The Most Wanted Healthy Diabetes Cookbook

Do Yourself a Big Favor with this Book

Evelin Turk

Table of Contents

Beef, Green Bean, And Basil Stir-fry

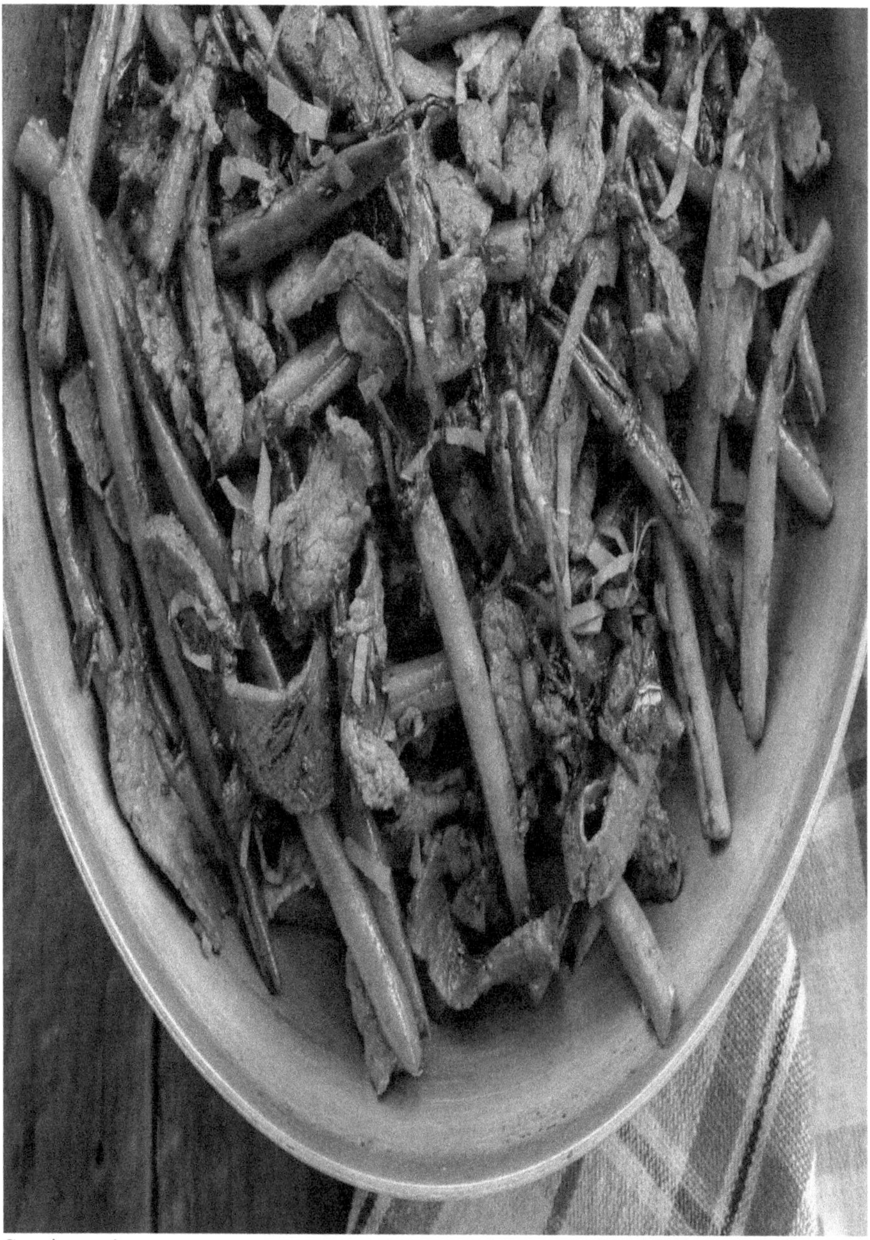

Servings: 4

Ingredients:

8 ounces green beans, trimmed

1⁄3 cup Chicken Stock or low-sodium chicken broth

2 tablespoons reduced-sodium soy sauce

1 tablespoon cornstarch

1⁄4 teaspoon chili-garlic paste

6 teaspoons canola oil, divided

1-pound top sirloin or flank steak, trimmed of all visible fat and cut into 1⁄4-inch-thick slices

2 garlic cloves, minced

1 small yellow bell pepper, thinly sliced

1 small red onion, halved lengthwise and thinly sliced

1⁄4 cup chopped fresh basil

Directions:

1. Fill a medium saucepan half full with water and bring to a boil over high heat. Add the green beans, return to a boil, and cook just until crisp-tender, about 3 minutes. Drain, let cool slightly, and pat dry with paper towels.
2. Combine the stock, soy sauce, cornstarch, and chili-garlic paste in a small bowl and stir until the cornstarch dissolves.
3. Heat a large wok or nonstick skillet over medium-high heat. Add 2 teaspoons of the oil and tilt the pan to coat the bottom evenly. Add half of the beef and cook, stirring constantly, until lightly browned, 2 to 3 minutes. Transfer the beef to a plate. Repeat with 2 teaspoons of the remaining oil and the remaining beef.
4. Wipe out the wok with paper towels. Add the remaining 2 teaspoons oil to the wok over medium-high heat. Add the garlic and cook, stirring constantly, until fragrant, 30 seconds. Add the green beans, bell pepper, and onion and cook, stirring constantly, until crisp-tender, 5 minutes. Stir in the beef and the stock mixture and cook, stirring constantly, until the sauce is thickened, 30 seconds. Remove from the heat and stir in the basil. Divide evenly among 4 plates and serve at once.

Nutrition Info:

10 g carb, 265 cal, 13 g fat, 2 g sat fat, 46 mg chol, 3 g fib, 27 g pro, 380 mg sod • Carb Choices: 1⁄2; Exchanges: 2 veg, 3 lean protein, 1 1⁄2 fat

Perfect-every-time Beef Tenderloin

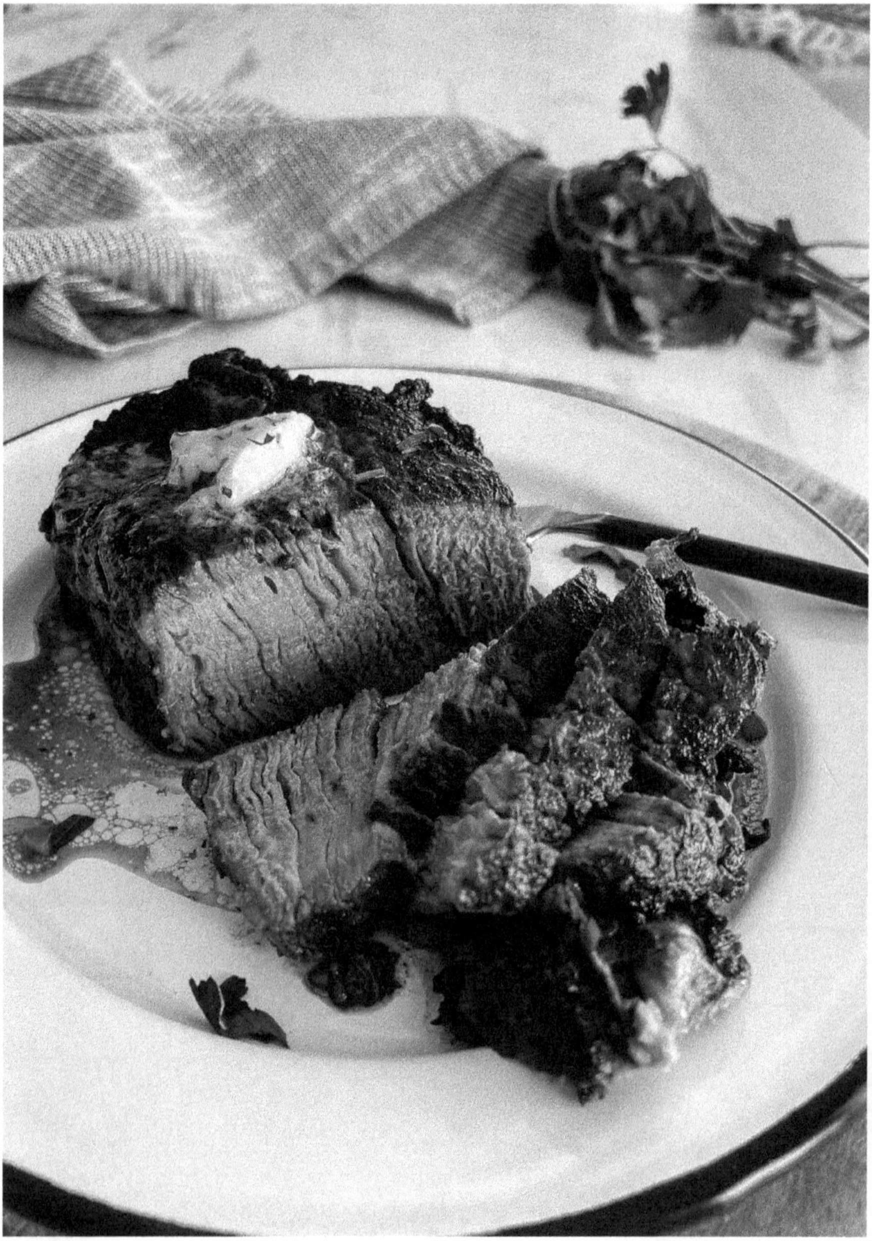

Servings: 8

Ingredients:

1 (2-pound) beef tenderloin, trimmed of all visible fat

1 teaspoon kosher salt

1/2 teaspoon freshly ground pepper

2 teaspoons extra virgin olive oil

Directions:

1. Preheat the oven to 400°F.
2. Sprinkle the tenderloin with the salt and pepper. Heat a large heavy- bottomed ovenproof skillet over medium-high heat. Add the oil and tilt the pan to coat the bottom evenly. Add the tenderloin and cook, turning to brown all sides, about 5 minutes.
3. Transfer the skillet to the oven and bake until an instant-read thermometer inserted into the center of the tenderloin reads 145°F about 15 minutes. Transfer the tenderloin to a cutting board, cover loosely with foil, and let stand about 10 minutes. Cut into slices, divide evenly among 8 plates, and serve at once.

Nutrition Info:

0 g carb, 187 cal, 9 g fat, 3 g sat fat, 79 mg chol, 0 g fib, 25 g pro, 190 mg sod • Carb Choices: 0; Exchanges: 3 lean protein

Beef, Cheddar, And Black Bean Burgers

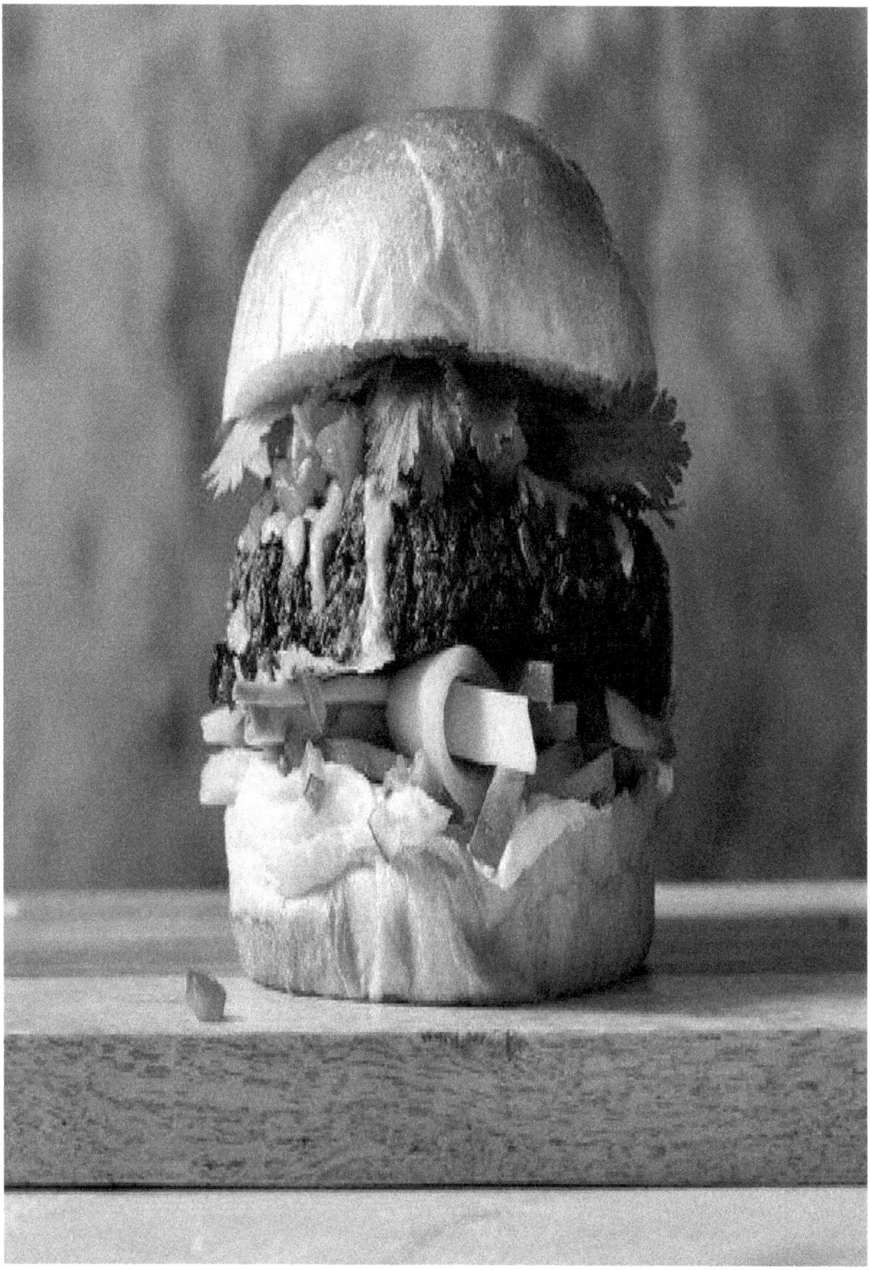

Servings: 4

Ingredients:

1 cup canned no-salt-added black beans, rinsed and drained

12 ounces 95% lean ground beef

2 tablespoons shredded reduced-fat extra-sharp Cheddar cheese

1⁄4 cup plain dry breadcrumbs

1⁄4 cup chopped fresh cilantro

1 jalapeño, seeded and minced

2 teaspoons chili powder

1 teaspoon ground cumin

1⁄2 teaspoon kosher salt

1⁄8 teaspoon freshly ground pepper

2 teaspoons canola oil

4 whole wheat sandwich rolls, toasted

1 medium tomato, sliced

4 large leaves leaf lettuce

Directions:

1. Place the beans in a large bowl and mash with a potato masher. Add the beef, Cheddar, breadcrumbs, cilantro, jalapeño, chili powder, cumin, salt, and pepper and mix thoroughly with your hands. Shape into 4 patties.
2. Heat a large nonstick skillet over medium heat. Add the oil and tilt the pan to coat the bottom evenly. Add the patties and cook, turning once, 4 minutes on each side for medium, or to the desired degree of doneness. Serve the patties in the rolls, topped with the tomato and lettuce.

Nutrition Info:

38 g carb, 340 cal, 9 g fat, 2 g sat fat, 49 mg chol, 7 g fib, 26 g pro, 532 mg sod • Carb Choices: 2; Exchanges: 11⁄2 starch, 1⁄2 carb, 3 lean protein, 1 fat

Two-bean Minestrone

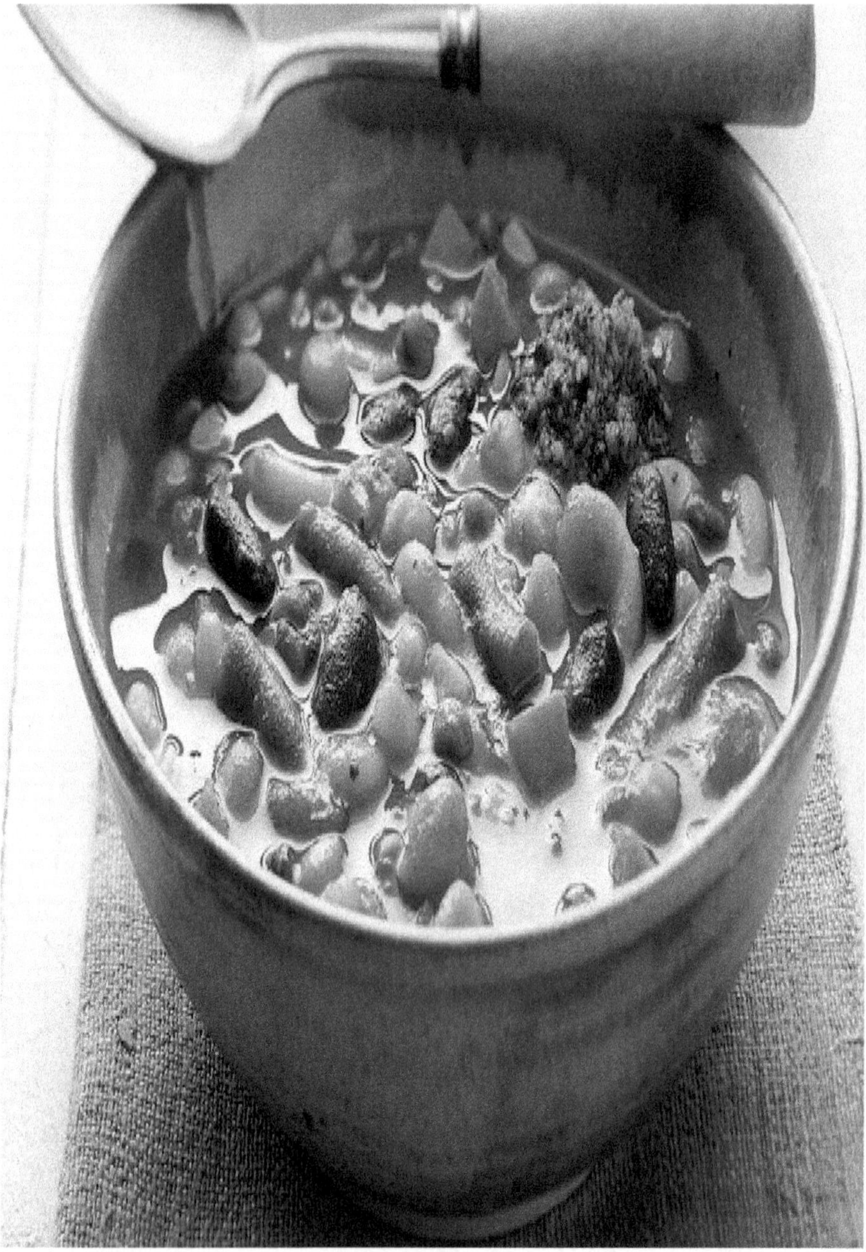

Servings: 8

Ingredients:

21⁄4 ounces whole wheat macaroni (about 3⁄4 cup)

2 teaspoons extra virgin olive oil

2 carrots, peeled and chopped

1 stalk celery, chopped

1 medium onion, chopped

2 garlic cloves, minced

6 cups Vegetable Stock or low-sodium vegetable broth

1 (141⁄2-ounce) can no-salt-added diced tomatoes

1⁄4 cup no-salt-added tomato paste

1⁄2 teaspoon kosher salt

1 teaspoon dried basil

1⁄2 teaspoon dried oregano

1⁄4 teaspoon freshly ground pepper-

1 (15-ounce) can no-salt-added garbanzo beans, rinsed and drained

1 cup frozen shelled edamame or frozen baby lima beans

1 medium zucchini, cut in half lengthwise and sliced

4 cups chopped fresh spinach

4 tablespoons freshly grated Parmesan

Directions:

1. Cook the macaroni according to the package directions.
2. Meanwhile, heat a large pot over medium heat. Add the oil and tilt the pot to coat the bottom evenly. Add the carrots, celery, and onion and cook, stirring often, until the vegetables are softened, 5 minutes. Stir in the garlic and cook, stirring constantly, until fragrant, 30 seconds.
3. Add the stock, tomatoes, tomato paste, salt, basil, oregano, and pepper and bring to a boil over high heat. Cover, reduce the heat to low, and simmer until the vegetables are tender, about 20 minutes.
4. Add the garbanzo beans, edamame, and zucchini and cook until the zucchini is crisp-tender, about 5 minutes. Turn off the heat and stir in the spinach and macaroni. Ladle the soup into 8 bowls, sprinkle evenly with the Parmesan, and serve at once. The soup is best on the day it is made, but it can be refrigerated, covered, for up to 2 days.

Nutrition Info:

29 g carb, 180 cal, 3 g fat, 1 g sat fat, 2 mg chol, 6 g fib, 9 g pro, 367 mg sod • Carb Choices: 2; Exchanges: 1 starch, 1⁄2 carb, 1 veg, 1 plant-based protein

Blueberry-nectarine Crisp with Cornmeal-pecan Topping

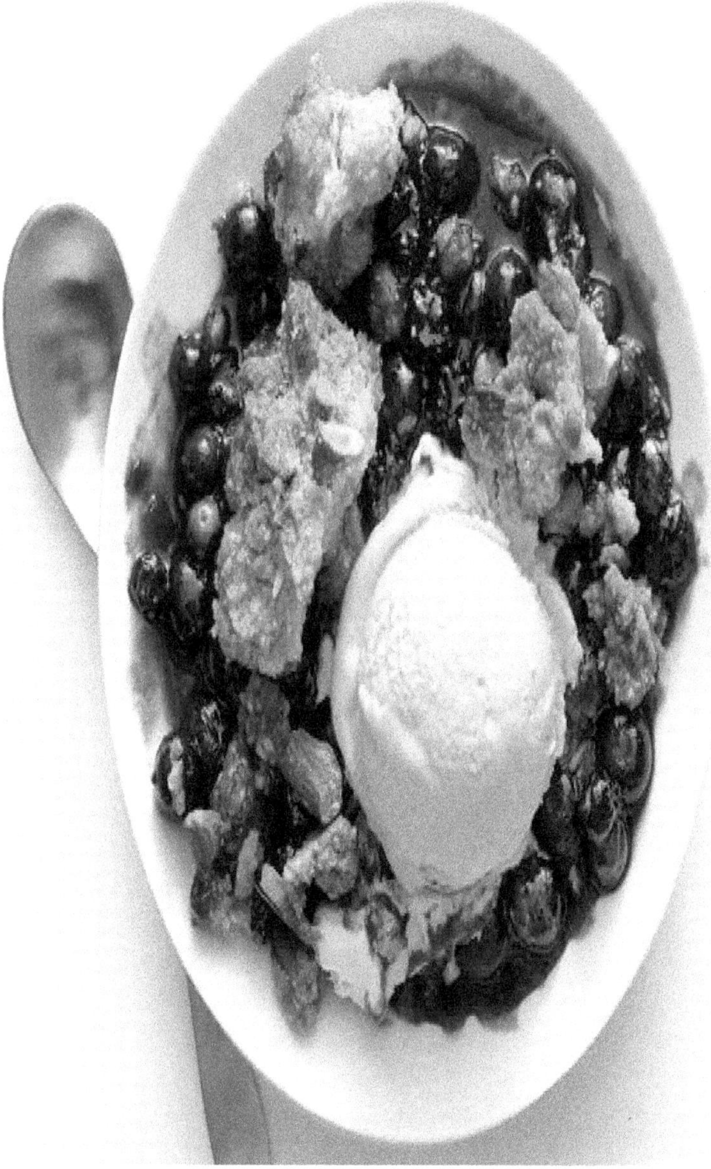

Servings: 8

Ingredients:

1 teaspoon canola oil

1⁄4 cup yellow cornmeal

1⁄4 cup packed light brown sugar

2 tablespoons cold unsalted butter, cut into small pieces

1⁄2 teaspoon ground cinnamon

1⁄4 cup chopped pecans

3 cups fresh blueberries or unthawed frozen blueberries

3 medium nectarines (about 1 1⁄4 pounds), pitted and sliced (about 3 cups)

2 tablespoons unbleached all-purpose flour

2 teaspoons grated lemon zest

Directions:

1. Preheat the oven to 350°F. Brush an 8-inch square baking dish with the oil.
2. Combine the cornmeal, sugar, butter, and cinnamon in a medium bowl. Using your fingers, blend the butter evenly into the cornmeal mixture. Add the pecans and set aside.
3. Combine the blueberries, nectarines, flour, and lemon zest in a large bowl and toss to combine. Spoon the blueberry mixture into the prepared dish. Sprinkle the cornmeal topping mixture over the blueberry mixture.
4. Bake until the topping is lightly browned and the fruit is bubbly around the edges, 25 to 30 minutes. Let stand 10 minutes before serving. Serve warm.

Nutrition Info:

26 g carb, 160 cal, 7 g fat, 2 g sat fat, 8 mg chol, 3 g fib, 2 g pro, 5 mg sod • Carb Choices: 2; Exchanges: 1 1/2 carb, 1/2 fruit, 1 fat

Bean And Vegetable Stew with Crispy Breadcrumbs

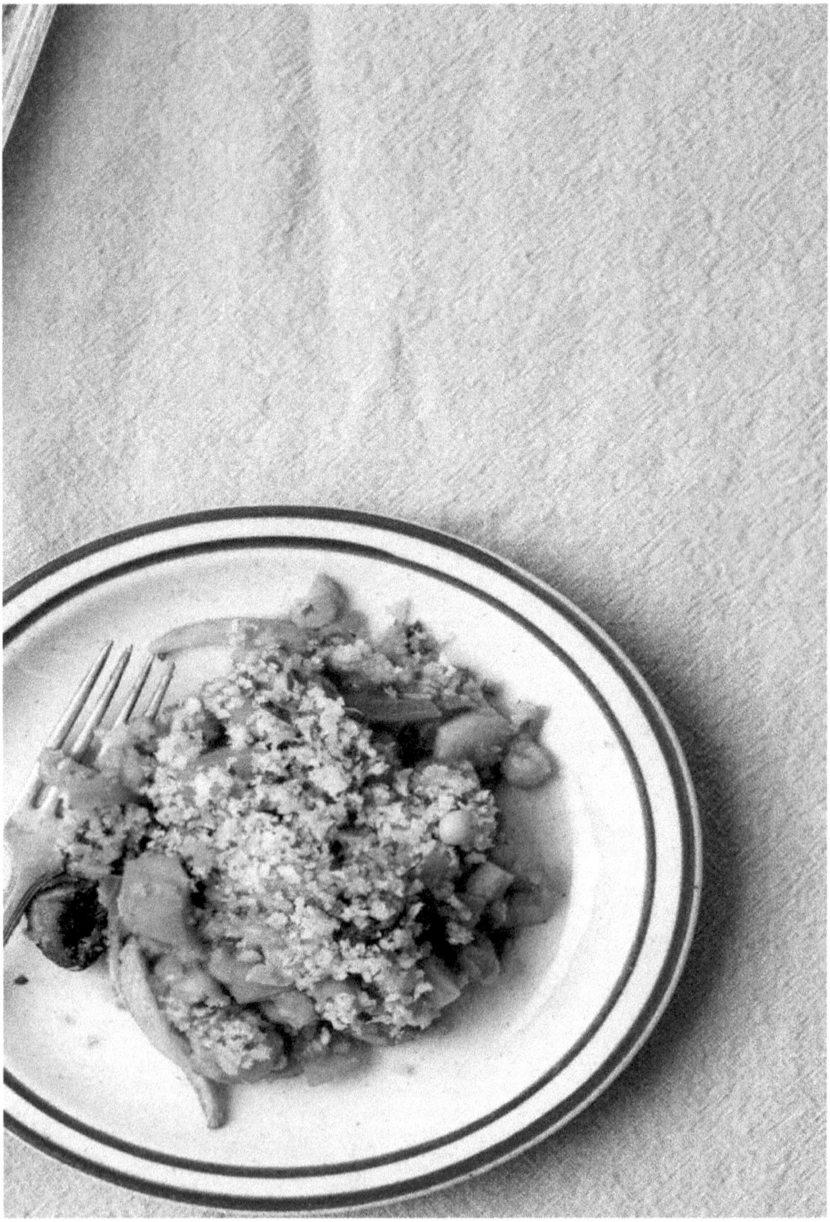

Servings: 4

Ingredients:

4 teaspoons extra virgin olive oil, divided

1 large onion, chopped

2 garlic cloves, minced

2 carrots, peeled and chopped

1 stalk celery, chopped

1 medium turnip, peeled and chopped

2 (15-ounce) cans no-salt-added navy beans, rinsed and drained

1 1/2 cups Vegetable Stock or low-sodium vegetable broth

2 tablespoons no-salt-added tomato paste

1/2 teaspoon kosher salt

1/4 teaspoon freshly ground pepper

3/4 cup fresh whole wheat breadcrumbs

1 garlic clove, crushed through a press

4 plum tomatoes, chopped

2 tablespoons chopped fresh basil

Directions:

1. Heat a large pot over medium-high heat. Add 2 teaspoons of the oil and tilt the pot to coat the bottom evenly. Add the onion and cook, stirring often, until the onion is softened, 5 minutes. Stir in the garlic and cook, stirring constantly, until fragrant, 30 seconds.
2. Add the carrots, celery, turnip, beans, stock, tomato paste, salt, and pepper and bring to a boil over high heat. Cover, reduce the heat to low, and simmer until the vegetables are very tender, about 15 minutes.
3. Preheat the oven to 350°F.
4. Stir together the breadcrumbs, garlic, and the remaining 2 teaspoons oil in a small bowl until the crumbs are moist. Place the crumbs in a small rimmed baking sheet and bake, stirring once, until crisp, 8 to 10 minutes.
5. Add the tomatoes to the stew and cook just until heated through, about 2 minutes. Remove the stew from the heat and stir in the basil. Ladle the stew into 4 bowls, sprinkle evenly with the crumbs, and serve at once. The stew can be refrigerated, covered, for up to 4 days.

Nutrition Info:

32 g carb, 228 cal, 6 g fat, 1 g sat fat, 0 mg chol, 10 g fib, 9 g pro, 303 mg sod • Carb Choices: 2; Exchanges: 11⁄2 starch, 1 veg, 1 plant- based protein, 1 fat

Guacamole

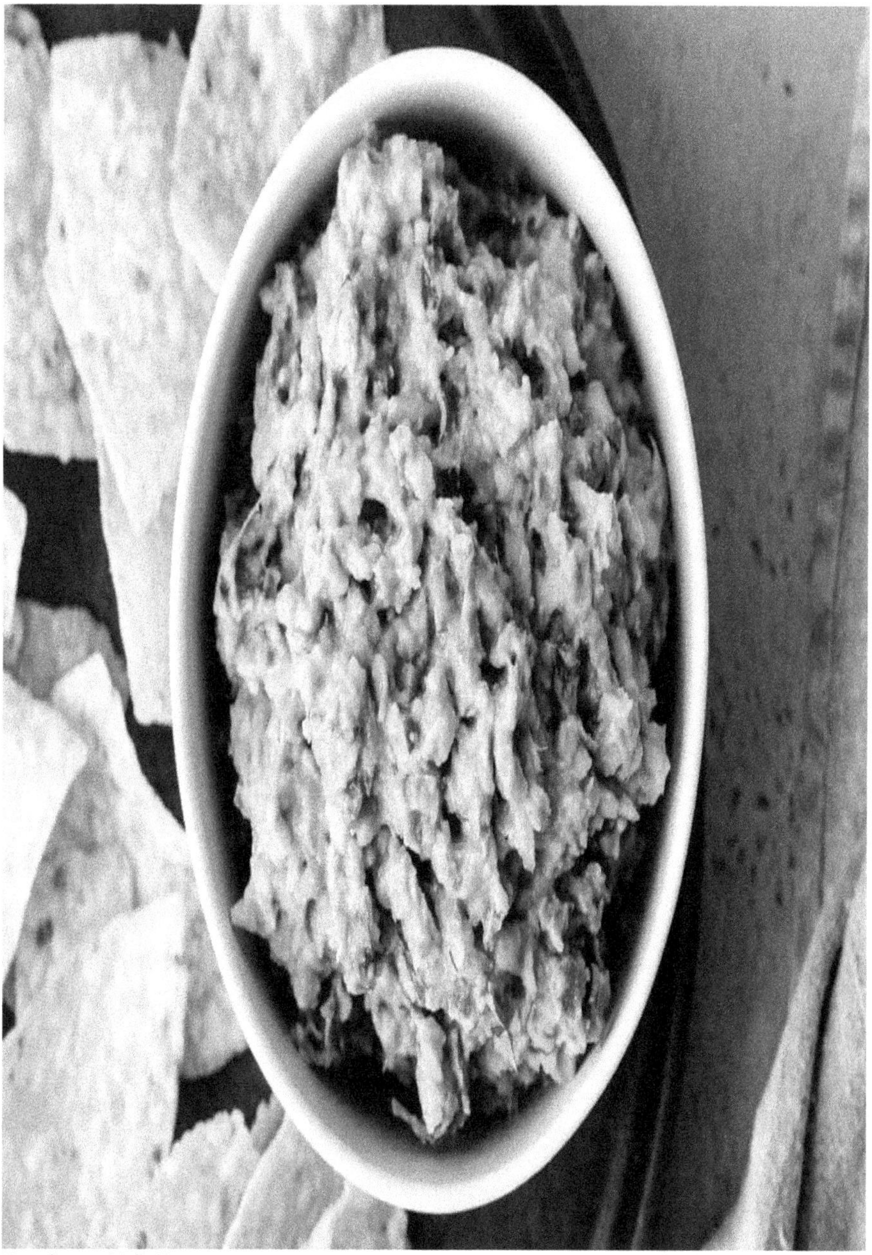

Servings: 11⁄2 Cups

Ingredients:

1 ripe Hass avocado, pitted, peeled, and chopped

1 large plum tomato, chopped

2 tablespoons minced red onion

2 tablespoons chopped fresh cilantro

1 tablespoon lime juice

1 garlic clove, crushed through a press

1⁄2 jalapeño, seeded and minced

1⁄2 teaspoon kosher salt

Directions:

1. Place the avocado in a medium bowl and gently mash with a spatula or fork until the avocado is creamy, but still chunky. Add the tomato, onion, cilantro, lime juice, garlic, jalapeño, and salt and stir to combine. Serve at once, or cover the surface of the guacamole with wax paper to prevent browning and refrigerate up to 4 hours.

Nutrition Info:

6 g carb, 88 cal, 7 g fat, 1 g sat fat, 0 mg chol, 4 g fib, 1 g pro, 145 mg sod • Carb Choices: 1⁄2; Exchanges: 1⁄2 carb, 1 1⁄2 fat

Orchard Spinach Salad with Toasted Almonds

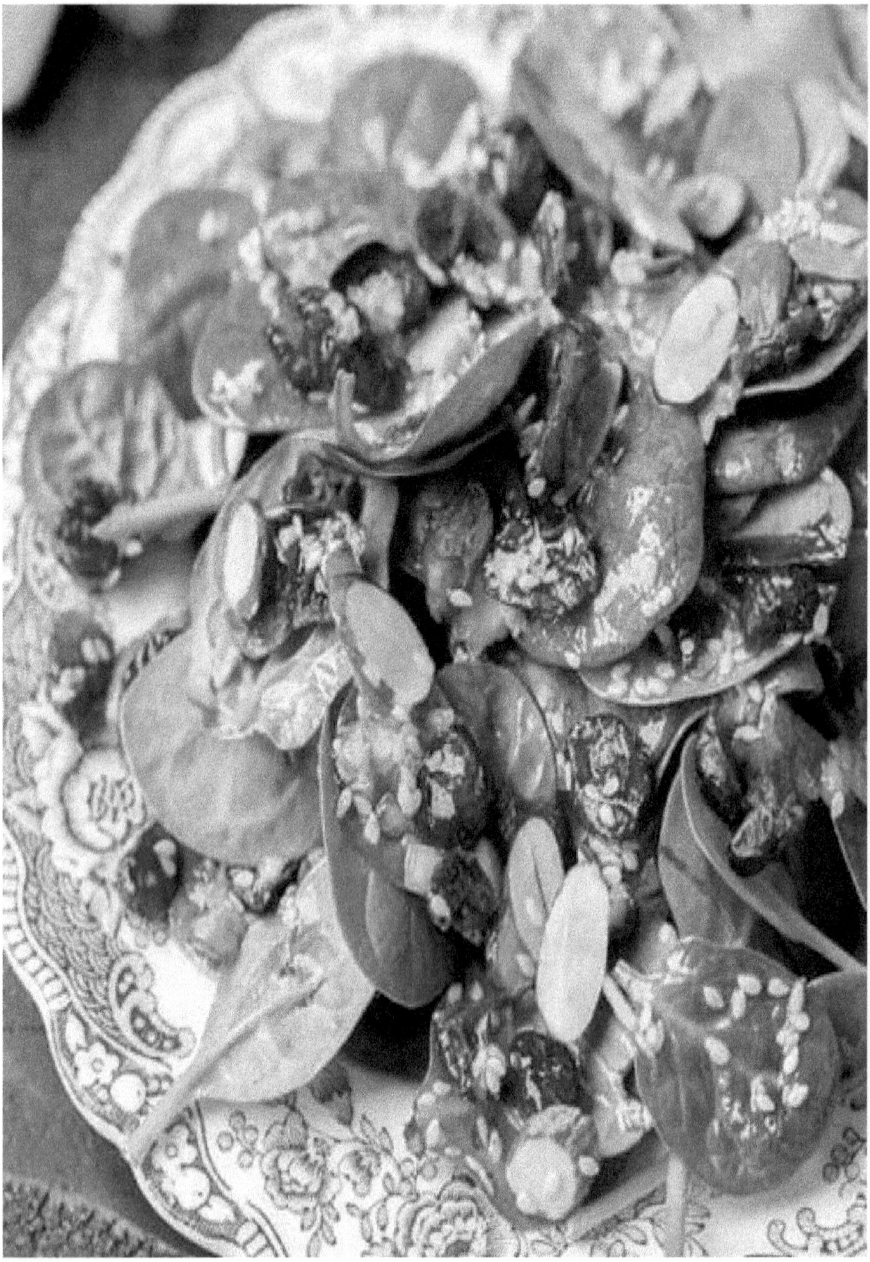

Servings: 4

Ingredients:

1⁄4 cup orange juice

2 dried apricots, chopped

1 tablespoon white wine vinegar

1 tablespoon extra virgin olive oil

1⁄2 teaspoon kosher salt

1⁄4 teaspoon freshly ground pepper

1 tablespoon minced red onion

8 cups loosely packed torn fresh spinach

1 apple, cored and thinly sliced

2 tablespoons golden raisins

2 tablespoons sliced almonds, toasted

Directions:

1. Pour the orange juice into a glass measuring cup. Add the apricots, cover with plastic wrap and microwave on high for 1 minute. Let cool slightly and place in a blender. Add the vinegar, oil, salt, and pepper and process until smooth. Transfer to a large bowl and stir in the onion.
2. Add the spinach, apple, raisins, and almonds and toss to coat. Serve at once.

Nutrition Info:

15 g carb, 111 cal, 5 g fat, 1 g sat fat, 0 mg chol, 3 g fib, 3 g pro, 189 mg sod • Carb Choices: 1; Exchanges: 1 fruit, 1 fat

Green Beans with Caramelized Onions And Cider Vinegar

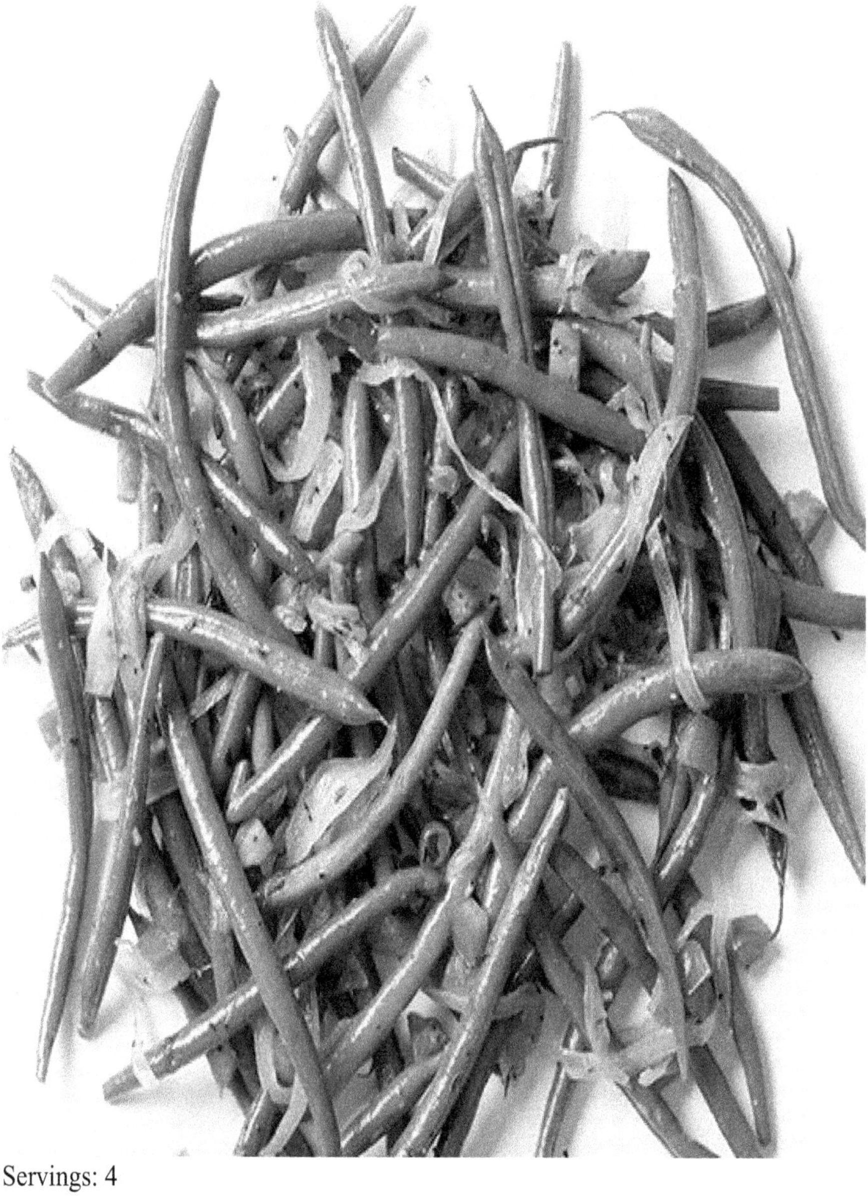

Servings: 4

Ingredients:

2 teaspoons extra virgin olive oil

1 medium onion, halved and thinly sliced

1-pound green beans, trimmed

2 teaspoons apple cider vinegar

1⁄2 teaspoon kosher salt

Pinch of freshly ground pepper

Directions:

1. Heat a medium nonstick skillet over medium heat. Add the oil and tilt the pan to coat the bottom evenly. Add the onion and cook, stirring often, until very soft and browned, about 20 minutes.
2. Meanwhile, in a saucepan fitted with a steamer basket, bring 1 inch of water to a boil over high heat. Add the green beans, reduce the heat to low, cover, and steam until tender, 4 to 5 minutes.
3. Add the green beans, vinegar, salt, and pepper to the onion and stir to combine. Spoon the green beans and onion into a serving dish and serve hot or warm.

Nutrition Info:

10 g carb, 63 cal, 3 g fat, 0 g sat fat, 0 mg chol, 4 g fib, 2 g pro, 147 mg sod • Carb Choices: 1⁄2; Exchanges: 2 veg, 1⁄2 fat

Rice with Tomato And Saffron

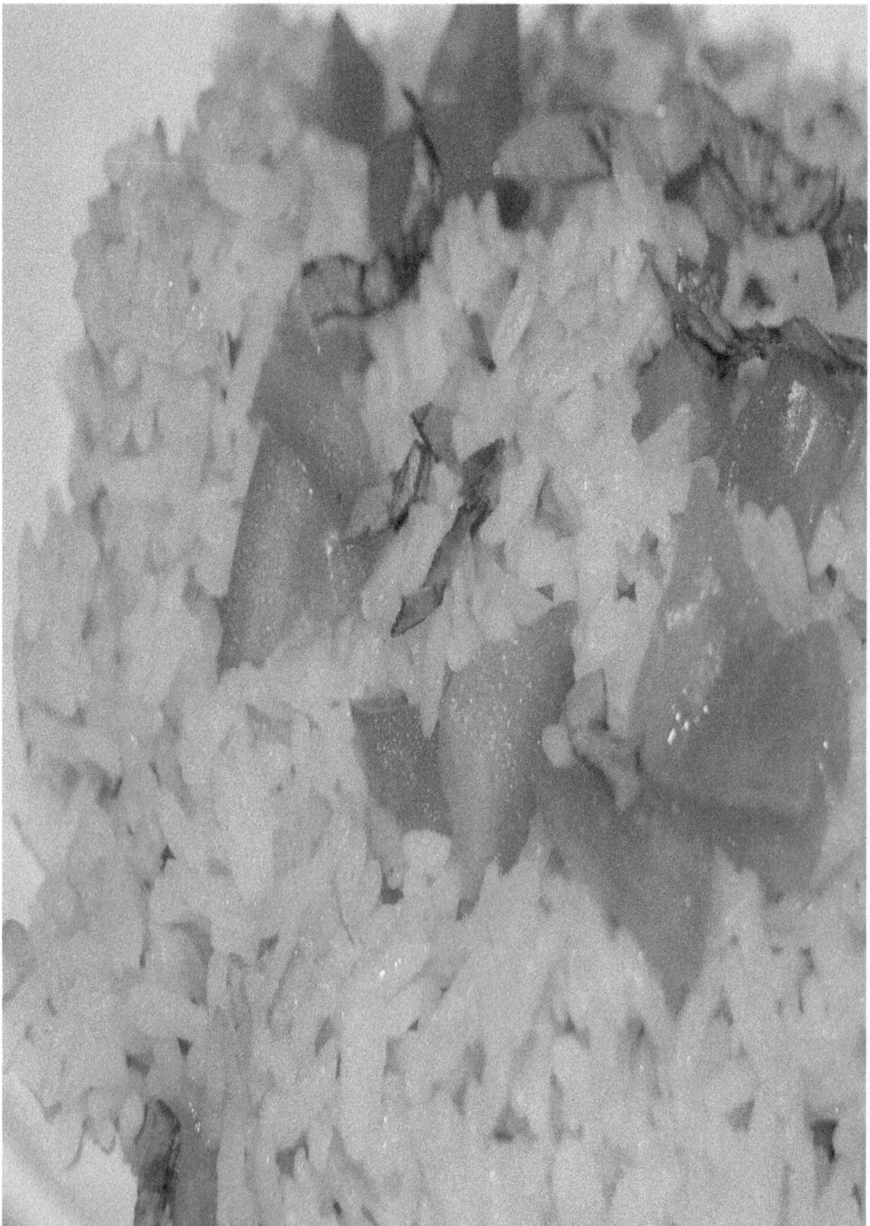

Servings: 4

Ingredients:

1⁄4 cup Vegetable Stock or low-sodium vegetable broth

Pinch of saffron threads

2 teaspoons extra virgin olive oil

1⁄4 cup diced onion

1⁄4 cup diced red bell pepper

1 garlic clove, minced

2 cups cooked brown rice

1 plum tomato, chopped

1⁄2 teaspoon kosher salt

Pinch of freshly ground pepper

1 tablespoon chopped fresh Italian parsley

Directions:

1. Pour the stock into a small bowl and microwave on high until hot, about 30 seconds. Add the saffron and set aside.
2. Heat a medium nonstick skillet over medium heat. Add the oil and tilt the pan to coat the bottom evenly. Add the onion and bell pepper and cook, stirring often, until softened, 5 minutes. Add the garlic and cook, stirring constantly, until fragrant, 30 seconds.
3. Add the stock mixture and bring to a boil over high heat. Reduce the heat to low and simmer, uncovered, until the vegetables are tender and most of the liquid has evaporated, about 3 minutes. Add the rice, tomato, salt, and ground pepper and cook, stirring often, until heated through, 2 minutes. Remove from the heat and stir in the parsley. Spoon the rice into a serving dish and serve at once.

Nutrition Info:

26 g carb, 142 cal, 3 g fat, 1 g sat fat, 0 mg chol, 2 g fib, 3 g pro, 152 mg sod • Carb Choices: 2; Exchanges: 2 starch, 1⁄2 fat

Spaghetti And Meatballs

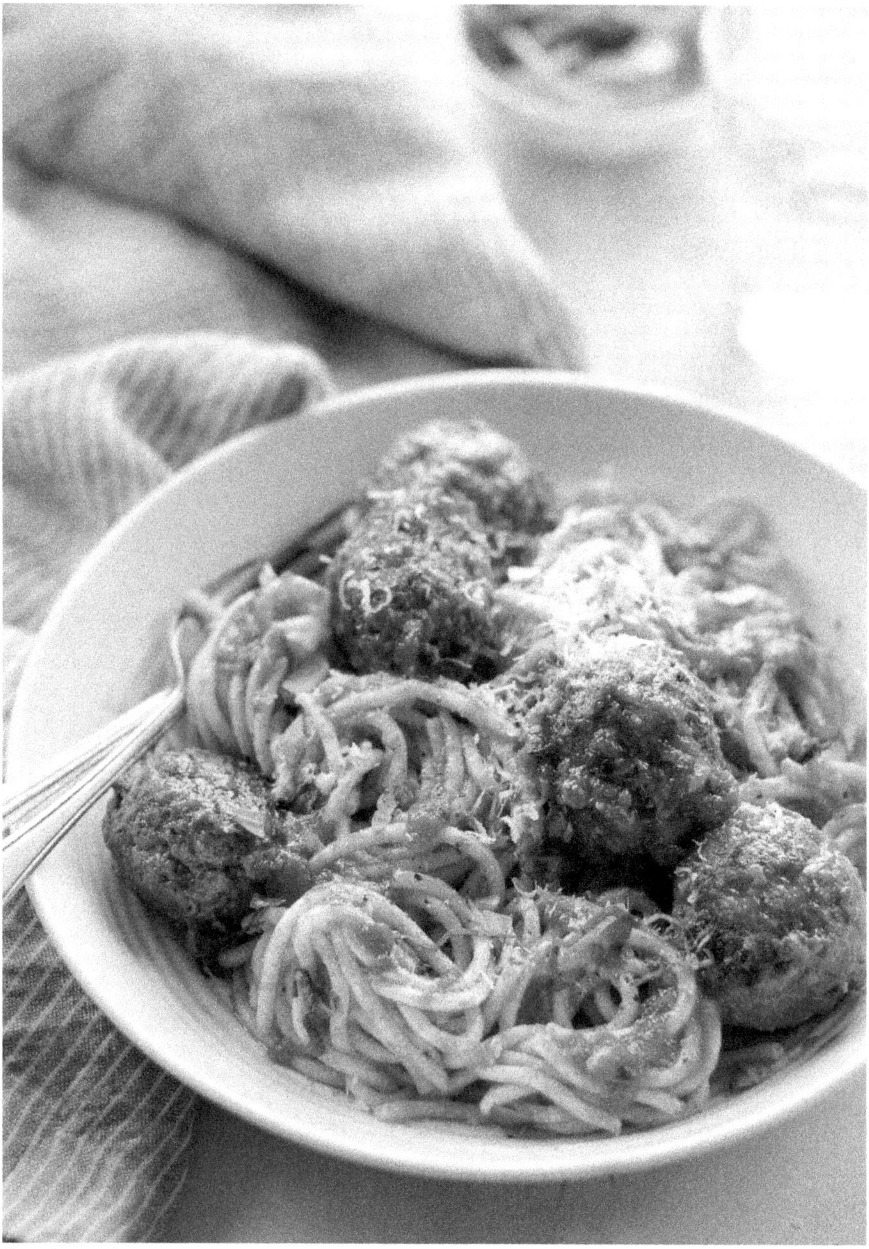

Servings: 4

Ingredients:

1 recipe Marinara Sauce

1⁄2 teaspoon canola oil

8 ounces Italian turkey sausage

8 ounces 95% lean ground beef

2 tablespoons minced onion

2 garlic cloves, minced

1 large egg white

2 tablespoons freshly grated Parmesan

1⁄4 cup plain dry breadcrumbs

1⁄4 cup chopped fresh Italian parsley

1⁄8 teaspoon freshly ground pepper

6 ounces whole wheat spaghetti

2 tablespoons finely shredded Parmesan

Directions:

1. Warm the sauce over medium heat, if necessary. Preheat the oven to 375°F. Line a large rimmed baking sheet with foil. Place a wire rack in the pan and brush the rack with the oil.
2. To make the meatballs, remove the sausage from the casings and place in a large bowl. Add the beef, onion, garlic, egg white, grated Parmesan, breadcrumbs, parsley, and pepper and mix thoroughly with your hands. Shape the mixture into about 32 (1-inch) meatballs and place on the prepared rack. Bake until the meatballs are lightly browned, about 20 minutes.
3. Transfer the meatballs to the pan of sauce. Simmer 5 minutes.
4. Meanwhile, cook the spaghetti according to the package directions. Divide the spaghetti evenly among 4 shallow bowls and top evenly with the meatballs and sauce. Sprinkle evenly with the shredded Parmesan and serve at once. You can make a double batch of the meatballs and sauce and freeze half for up to 3 months.

Nutrition Info:

58 g carb, 471 cal, 14 g fat, 3 g sat fat, 61 mg chol, 10 g fib, 33 g pro, 582 mg sod • Carb Choices: 3 1/2; Exchanges: 2 1/2 starch, 2 veg, 1 medium-fat protein, 1 1/2 lean protein, 1 fat

Mixed Tomato And Mozzarella Salad with Basil Dressing

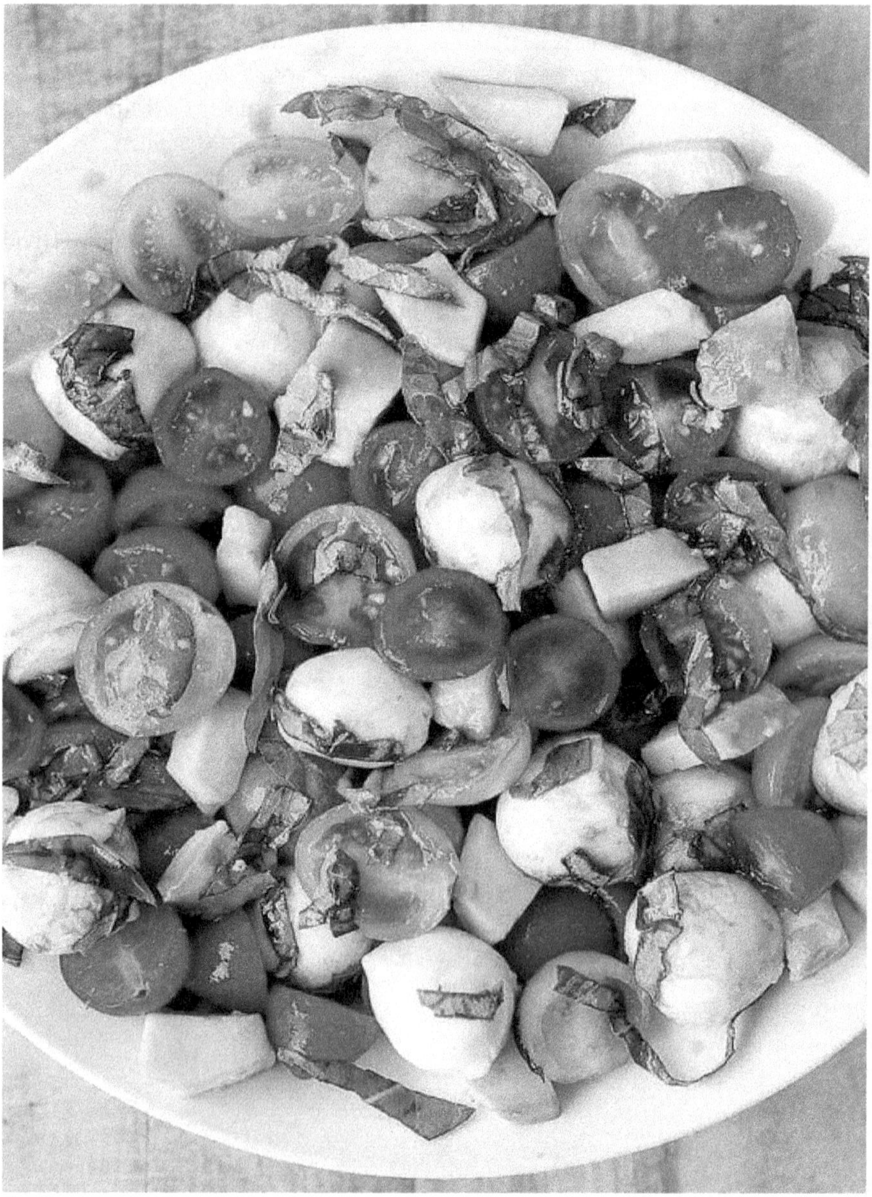

Servings: 8

Ingredients:

8 ounces fresh mozzarella, thinly sliced

4 large tomatoes, sliced

1 cup red cherry tomatoes, halved

1 cup yellow cherry tomatoes, halved

1 recipe Herbed Vinaigrette, made with fresh basil

Thinly sliced fresh basil leaves

Directions:

1. Arrange the mozzarella and sliced tomatoes in alternating layers on a large platter. Top with the cherry tomatoes. Drizzle with the vinaigrette and sprinkle with the basil. Serve at once.

Nutrition Info:

4 g carb, 139 cal, 12 g fat, 3 g sat fat, 10 mg chol, 1 g fib, 6 g pro, 69 mg sod • Carb Choices: 0; Exchanges: 1 veg, 1 medium-fat protein, 1 fat

Crispy Baked Root Vegetable Chips

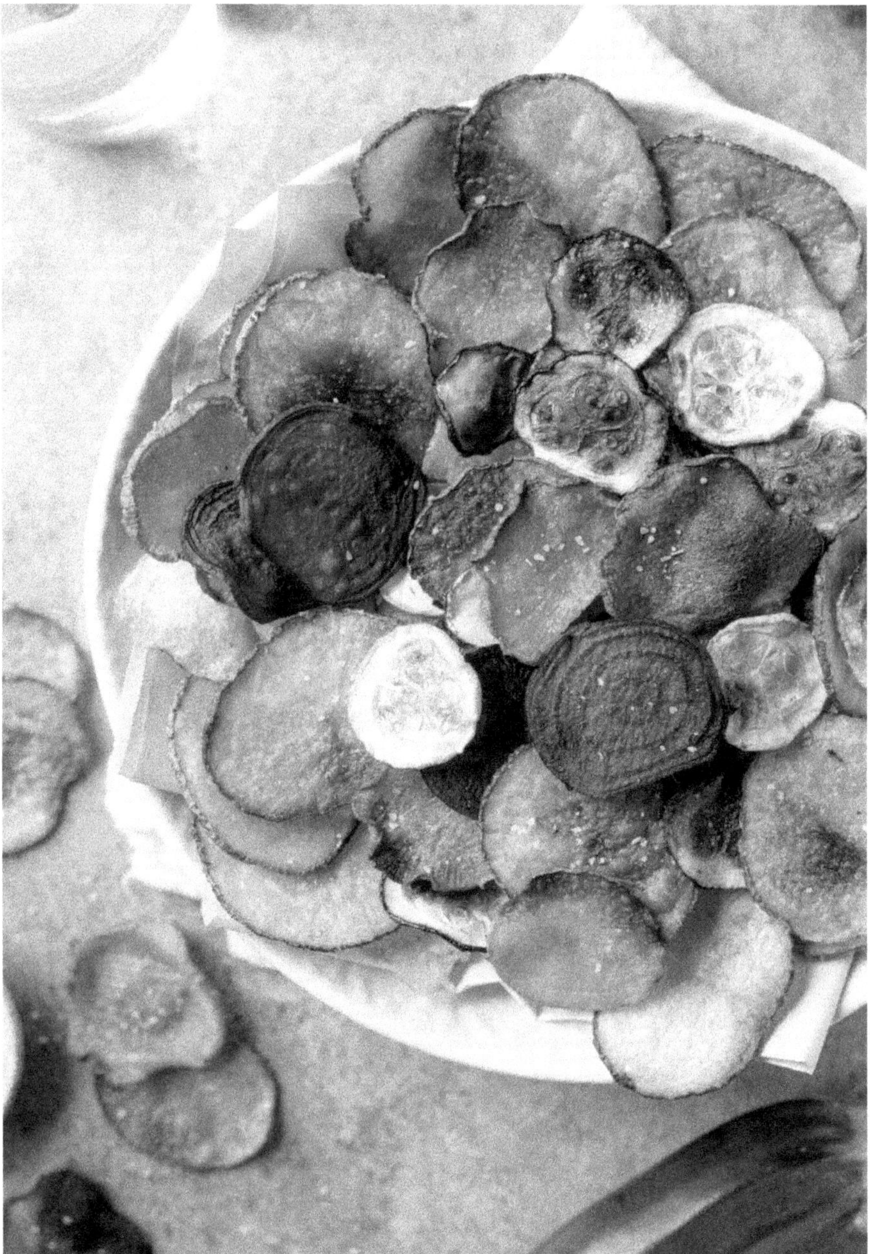

Servings: 4

Ingredients:

2 large carrots, peeled

1 small sweet potato, peeled

1 small baking potato, well scrubbed

2 teaspoons extra virgin olive oil

1⁄8 teaspoon salt

Directions:

1. Preheat the oven to 375°F.
2. Using the thin slicing blade on a food processor or a mandolin, cut the carrots and potatoes into 1/16-inch slices. Place the vegetables in a large bowl, drizzle with the oil, and toss to coat evenly.
3. Arrange the vegetables in a single layer on two large rimmed baking sheets. Bake until the chips are browned, 30 to 35 minutes, checking the chips often during the last 10 minutes of baking. Transfer the chips to a large bowl as they are done. Sprinkle the chips with the salt and toss to coat. The chips are best on the day they are made. If you do store them, they will likely lose their crispness. You can bake them on a baking sheet in a 250°F oven for 6 to 8 minutes to restore their crunch.

Nutrition Info:

14 g carb, 81 cal, 2 g fat, 0 g sat fat, 0 mg chol, 2 g fib, 2 g pro, 106 mg sod • Carb Choices: 1; Exchanges: 1 starch, 1/2 fat

Salmon with Warm Lentils

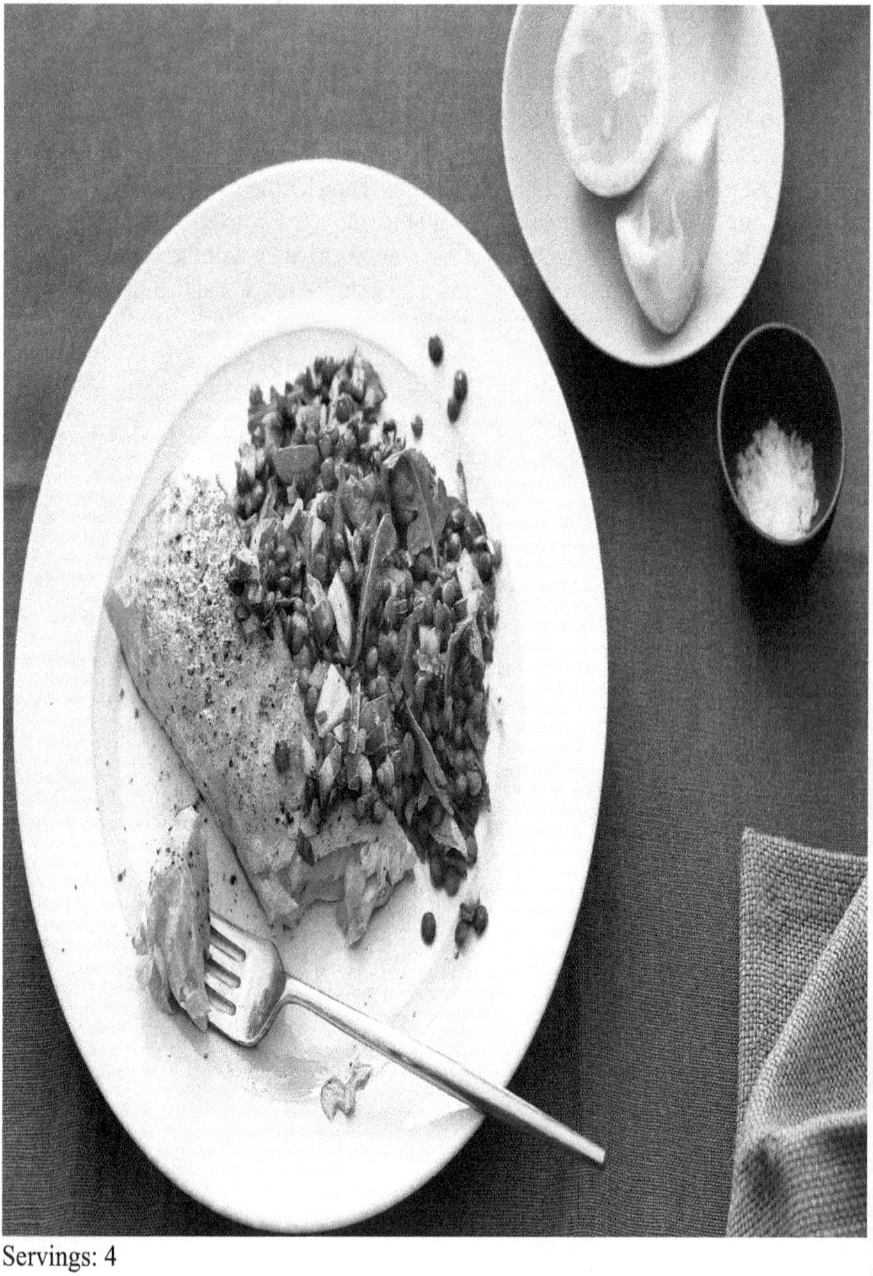

Servings: 4

Ingredients:

2 cups Chicken Stock or low-sodium chicken broth

1 cup dried French green lentils, picked over and rinsed

2 plum tomatoes, chopped

2 tablespoons diced red onion

1 tablespoon plus 2 teaspoons extra virgin olive oil, divided

1 tablespoon white wine vinegar

1⁄2 teaspoon kosher salt, divided

1⁄4 teaspoon freshly ground pepper, divided

4 (4-ounce) salmon fillets

1⁄4 cup chopped fresh Italian parsley

Directions:

1. Combine the stock and lentils in a medium saucepan. Bring to a boil over high heat. Cover, reduce the heat to low, and simmer until the lentils are tender but still retain their shape, 15 to 20 minutes. Drain and transfer to a medium bowl. Stir in the tomatoes, onion, 1 tablespoon of the oil, the vinegar, 1⁄4 teaspoon of the salt, and 1⁄8 teaspoon of the pepper. Let stand at room temperature while preparing the salmon.
2. Sprinkle the salmon with the remaining 1⁄4 teaspoon salt and remaining 1⁄8 teaspoon pepper. Heat a large nonstick skillet over medium-high heat. Add the remaining 2 teaspoons oil and tilt the pan to coat the bottom evenly. Add the salmon and cook, turning once, until the fish is opaque in the center, about 4 minutes on each side.
3. Stir the parsley into the lentil mixture. Spoon the lentils evenly onto 4 plates and top with the salmon. Serve at once.

Nutrition Info:

29 g carb, 406 cal, 15 g fat, 2 g sat fat, 74 mg chol, 8 g fib, 38 g pro, 267 mg sod • Carb Choices: 11⁄2; Exchanges: 11⁄2 starch, 4 lean protein, 1 plant-based protein, 1 fat

Crispy Tofu with Spicy Ginger-lime Soy Sauce

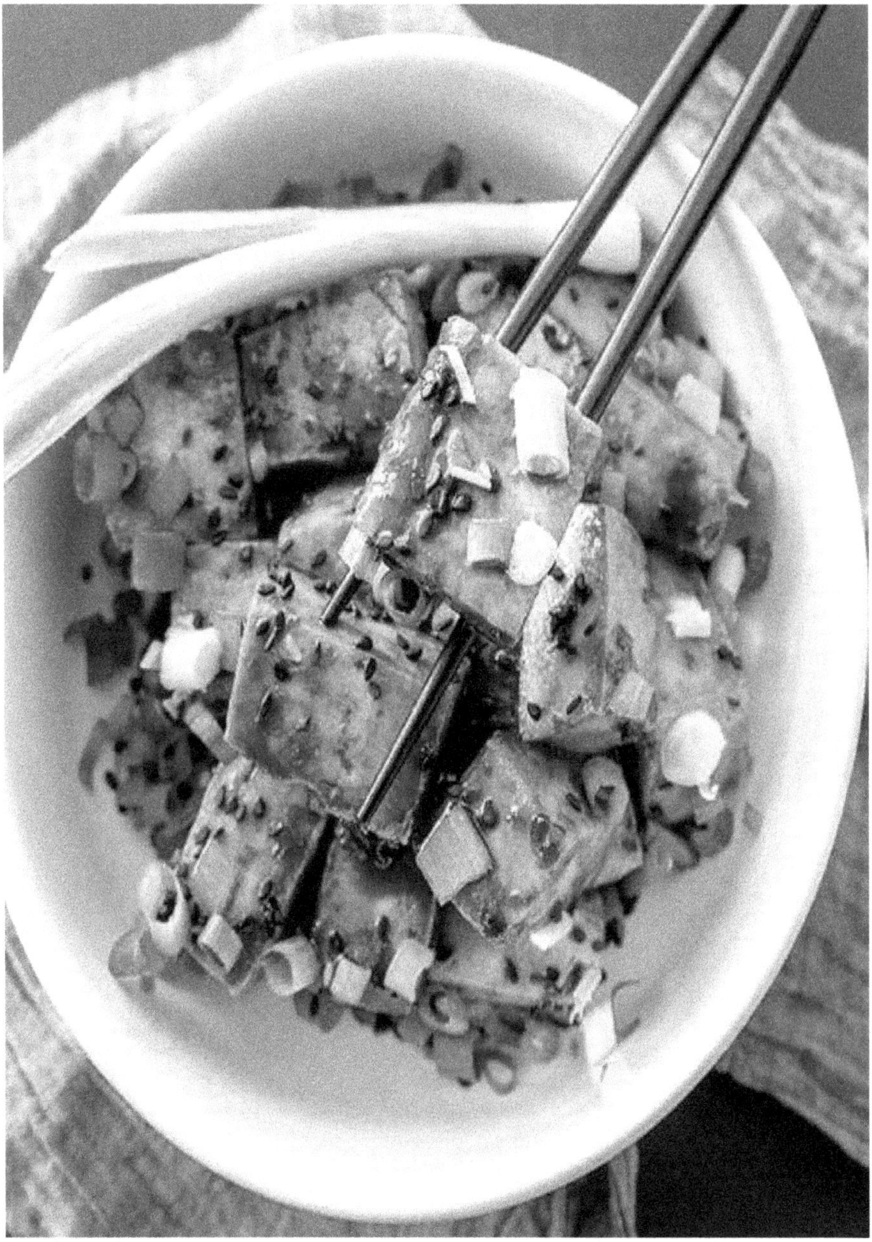

Servings: 4

Ingredients:

2 tablespoons reduced-sodium soy sauce

2 tablespoons lime juice

2 tablespoons water

2 teaspoons light brown sugar

1 teaspoon grated fresh ginger

1 teaspoon cornstarch

1⁄4 teaspoon chili-garlic paste

1 (1-pound) package extra-firm reduced-fat tofu

2 teaspoons canola oil

2 tablespoons chopped fresh cilantro

2 tablespoons thinly sliced scallion

Directions:

1. Combine the soy sauce, lime juice, water, sugar, ginger, cornstarch, and chili-garlic paste in a small saucepan and stir until the sugar dissolves. Set aside.
2. Cut the tofu in half lengthwise, then cut each piece in half crosswise. Pat dry with paper towels.
3. Heat a large wok or nonstick skillet over medium-high heat. Add the oil and tilt the pan to coat the bottom evenly. Add the tofu and cook, turning once, until well browned, 3 to 4 minutes on each side.
4. Meanwhile, set the soy sauce mixture over medium-high heat and cook, whisking often, until the mixture comes to a boil and thickens, about 3 minutes.
5. Place the tofu on a serving platter, drizzle with the sauce, and sprinkle with the cilantro and scallion. Divide the tofu and sauce evenly among 4 plates and serve at once.

Nutrition Info:

9 g carb, 153 cal, 7 g fat, 0 g sat fat, 0 mg chol, 3 g fib, 13 g pro, 311 mg sod • Carb Choices: 1⁄2; Exchanges: 1⁄2 carb, 2 plant-based protein, 1⁄2 fat

Blueberry-apricot Breakfast Casserole

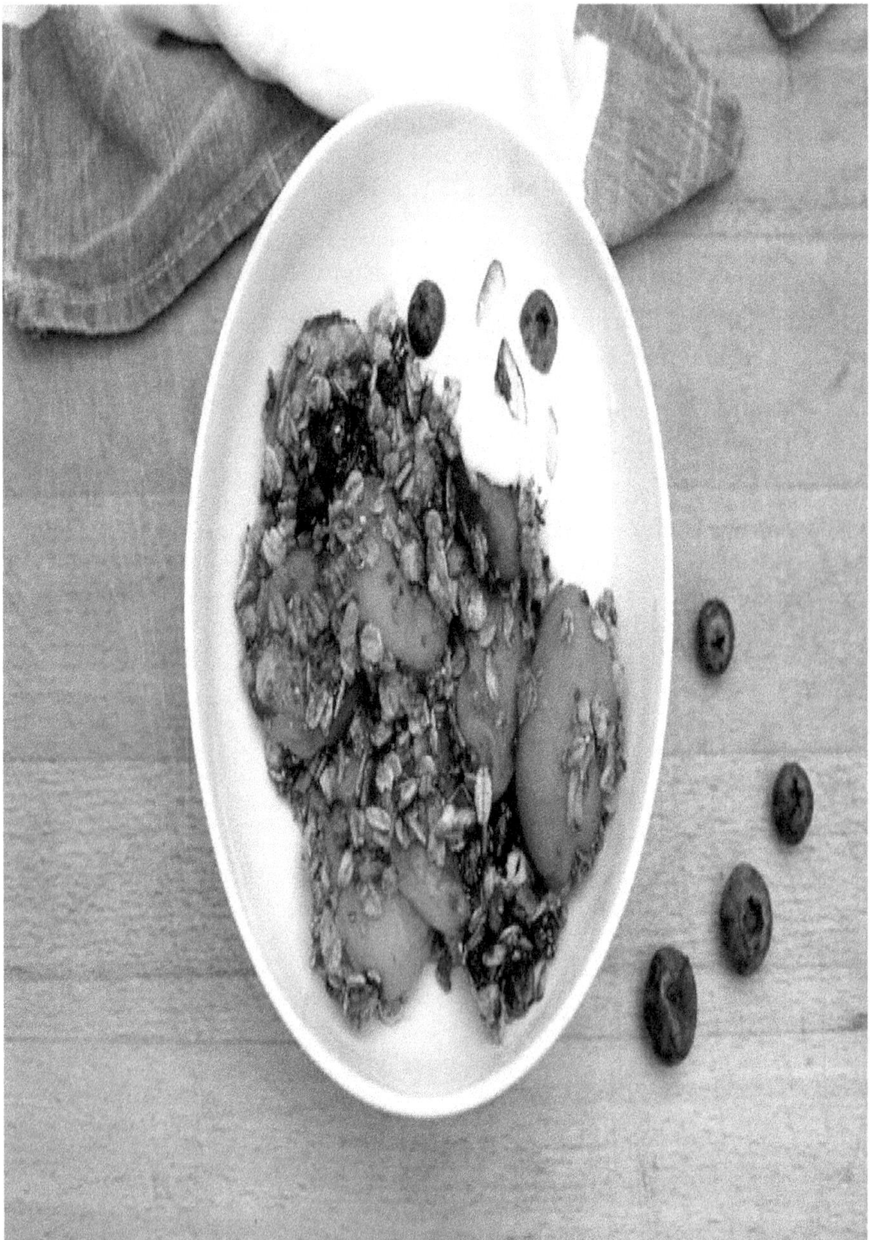

Servings: 6

Ingredients:

1 teaspoon canola oil

2 large eggs

4 large egg whites

1⁄2 cup 1% low-fat milk

1⁄3 cup apricot preserves

1⁄2 teaspoon vanilla extract

6 slices day-old 100% whole wheat bread, cut into 1⁄2-inch cubes (about 5 cups)

1 cup fresh blueberries

Directions:

1. Preheat the oven to 350°F. Preheat the oven to 350°F. Brush an 8-inch square baking pan with the oil.
2. Whisk together the eggs, egg whites, milk, preserves, and vanilla in a large bowl. Add the bread cubes and toss to combine. Let stand 5 minutes, tossing occasionally. Add the blueberries and toss to combine.
3. Spoon into the prepared baking dish. Bake, uncovered, until the top is lightly browned and the center is almost set, 30 to 35 minutes. Let stand 5 minutes before serving.

Nutrition Info:

32 g carb, 190 cal, 4 g fat, 1 g sat fat, 73 mg chol, 3 g fib, 9 g pro, 227 mg sod • Carb Choices: 2; Exchanges: 1 starch, 1 carb, 1 lean protein

Miso-vegetable Soup

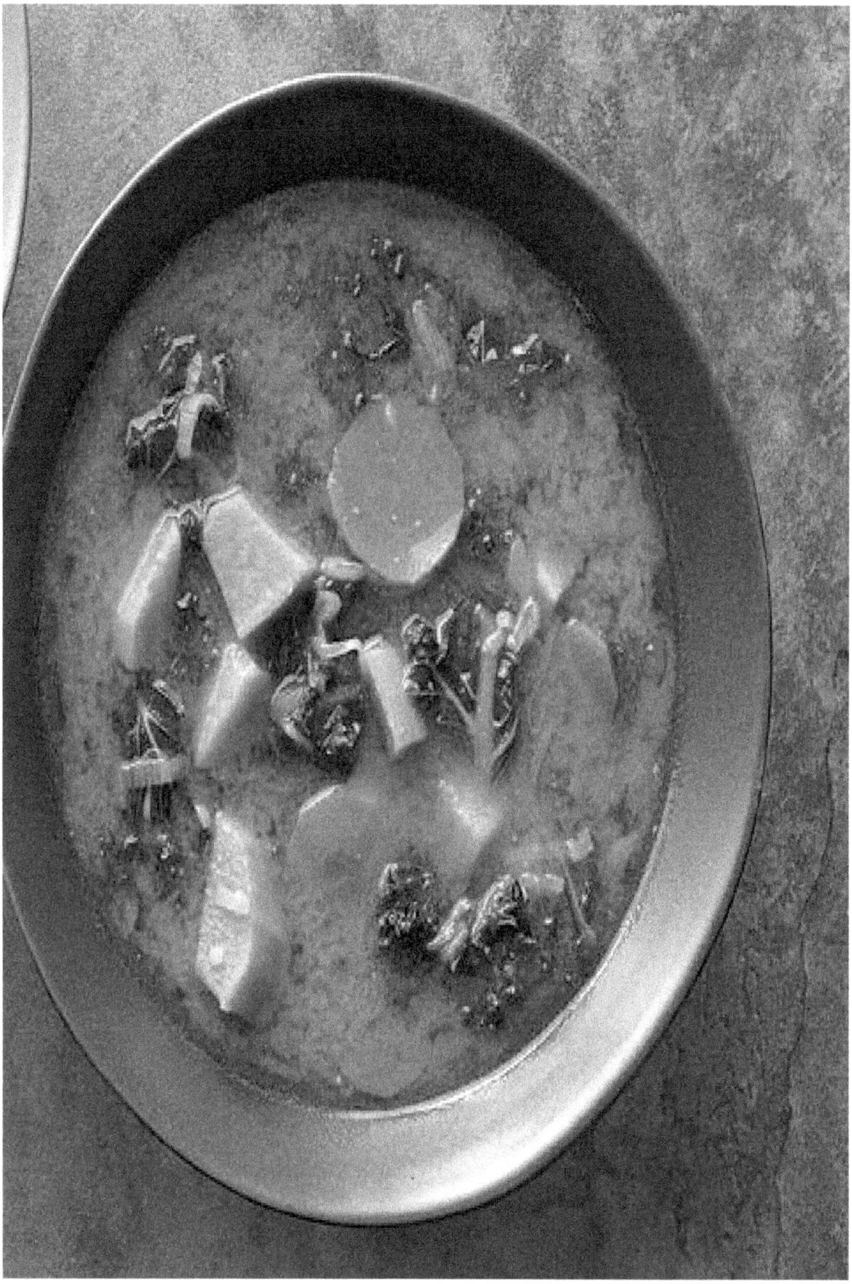

Servings: 6

Ingredients:

2 teaspoons canola oil

2 tablespoons minced fresh ginger

2 garlic cloves, minced

6 cups water

6 ounces shiitake mushrooms, stemmed and thinly sliced

4 ounces snow peas, trimmed and thinly sliced

2 medium carrots, peeled, cut in half lengthwise, and thinly sliced

1⁄3 cup white miso paste

1⁄2 teaspoon chili-garlic paste

1⁄2 teaspoon Asian sesame oil

Thinly sliced scallions

Chopped fresh cilantro

Directions:

1. Heat a large pot over medium heat. Add the canola oil and tilt the pan to coat the bottom evenly. Add the ginger and garlic and cook, stirring constantly, until fragrant, 30 seconds. Add the water and bring to a boil.
2. Add the mushrooms, snow peas, and carrots and return to a boil. Reduce the heat to low and simmer until the vegetables are crisp-tender, about 5 minutes. Ladle about 1 cup of the broth from the soup into a small bowl. Add the miso paste and whisk until the miso dissolves. Stir the miso mixture, chili-garlic paste, and sesame oil into the soup. Ladle the soup into 6 bowls, top each serving with the scallions and cilantro, and serve at once. The soup is best when eaten immediately.

Nutrition Info:

8 g carb, 66 cal, 2 g fat, 0 g sat fat, 0 mg chol, 2 g fib, 3 g pro, 685 mg sod • Carb Choices: 1⁄2; Exchanges: 1⁄2 carb

Cilantro Pesto

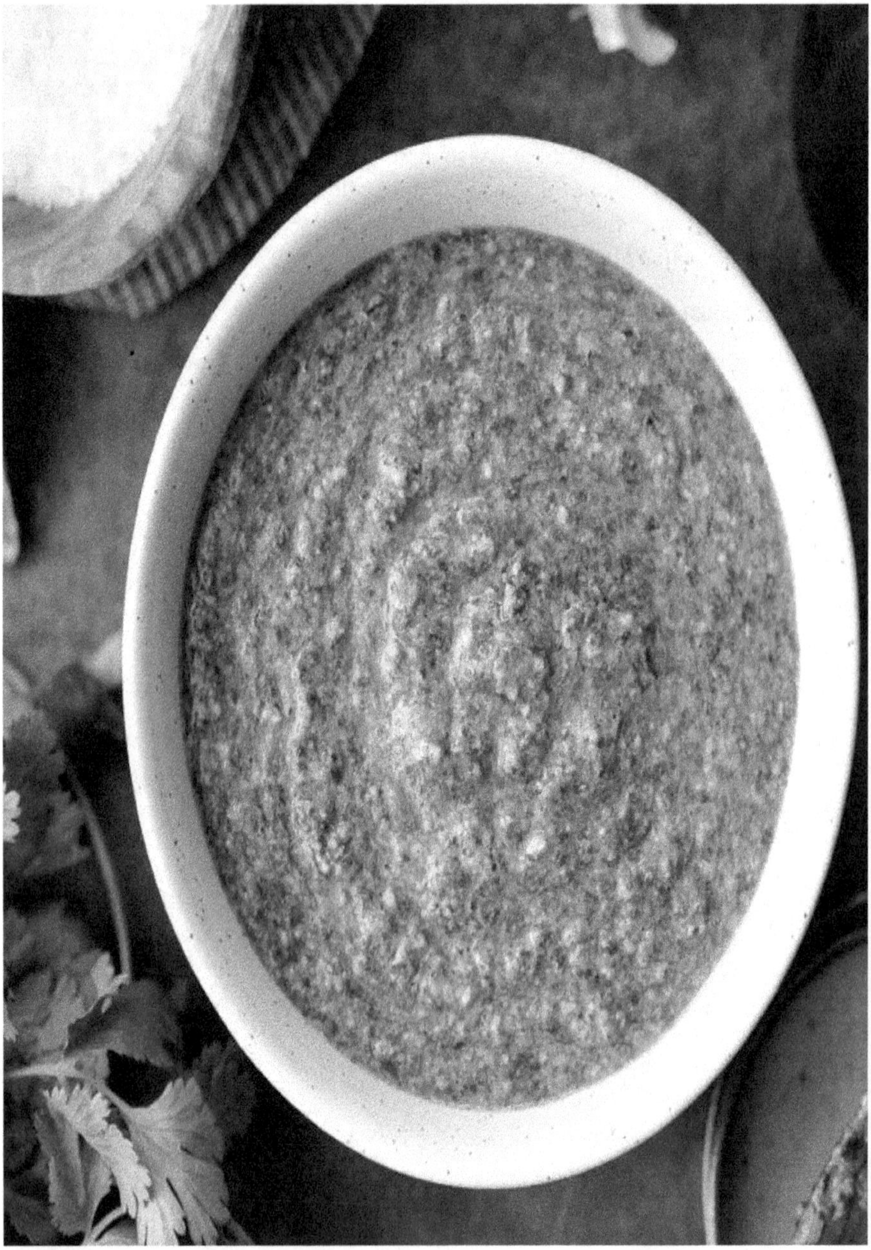

Servings: 1⁄2 Cup

Ingredients:

1⁄4 cup slivered almonds, toasted

1 cup tightly packed fresh cilantro leaves

1 ounce freshly grated Parmesan (about 1⁄4 cup)

3 tablespoons canola oil

1 tablespoon lime juice

1 small garlic clove, chopped

1⁄2 teaspoon ground cumin

1⁄4 teaspoon kosher salt

1⁄8 teaspoon ground cayenne

Directions:

1. Combine all the ingredients in a food processor and process until the mixture is finely chopped. The sauce can be refrigerated, with the surface covered with plastic wrap, for up to 4 days.

Nutrition Info:

1 g carb, 78 cal, 8 g fat, 1 g sat fat, 2 mg chol, 0 g fib, 2 g pro, 74 mg sod • Carb Choices: 0; Exchanges: 2 fat

Farro Risotto with Cherry Tomatoes, Feta, And Herbs

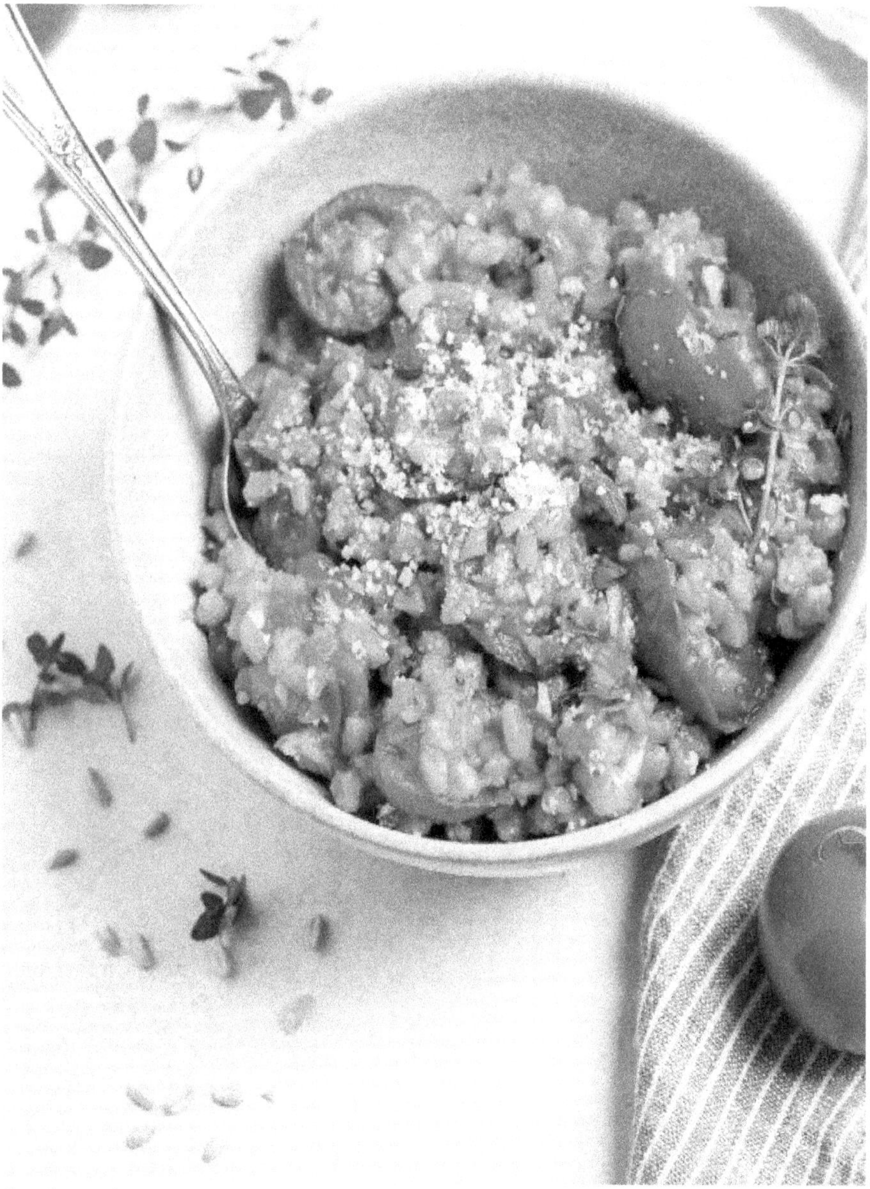

Servings: 6

Ingredients:

2 medium leeks, halved lengthwise and thinly sliced

4 cups Vegetable Stock or low-sodium vegetable broth

2 teaspoons extra virgin olive oil

1 cup farro

1⁄2 cup dry white wine

1⁄2 teaspoon kosher salt

3 cups cherry tomatoes, halved

2 ounces finely crumbled feta cheese (about 1⁄2 cup)

2 tablespoons any combination of chopped fresh basil, dill, mint, or Italian parsley

1 tablespoon lemon juice

Directions:

1. Submerge the sliced leeks in a large bowl of water, lift them out, and drain in a colander. Repeat, using fresh water, until no grit remains in the bottom of the bowl. Drain the leeks well.
2. Pour the stock into a medium saucepan and bring to a simmer over medium-high heat. Reduce the heat to low and keep the stock warm.
3. Heat a large saucepan over medium heat. Add the oil and tilt the pan to coat the bottom evenly. Add the leeks and cook, stirring often, until softened, 5 minutes.
4. Add the farro and cook, stirring constantly, 2 minutes. Add the wine and salt and cook, stirring frequently, until the liquid is absorbed. Add the stock, 1⁄2 cup at a time, and cook, stirring frequently, until the liquid is absorbed after each addition before adding more stock. When all the liquid is absorbed and the farro is tender, stir in the tomatoes, feta, and herbs and cook until the tomatoes are heated through, 2 minutes. Stir in the lemon juice. Divide among 6 bowls and serve at once.

Nutrition Info:

32 g carb, 214 cal, 4 g fat, 2 g sat fat, 8 mg chol, 5 g fib, 7 g pro, 302 mg sod • Carb Choices: 2; Exchanges: 1 1⁄2 starch, 1 veg, 1 fat

Grilled Marinated Lamb Chops with Orange-mint Relish

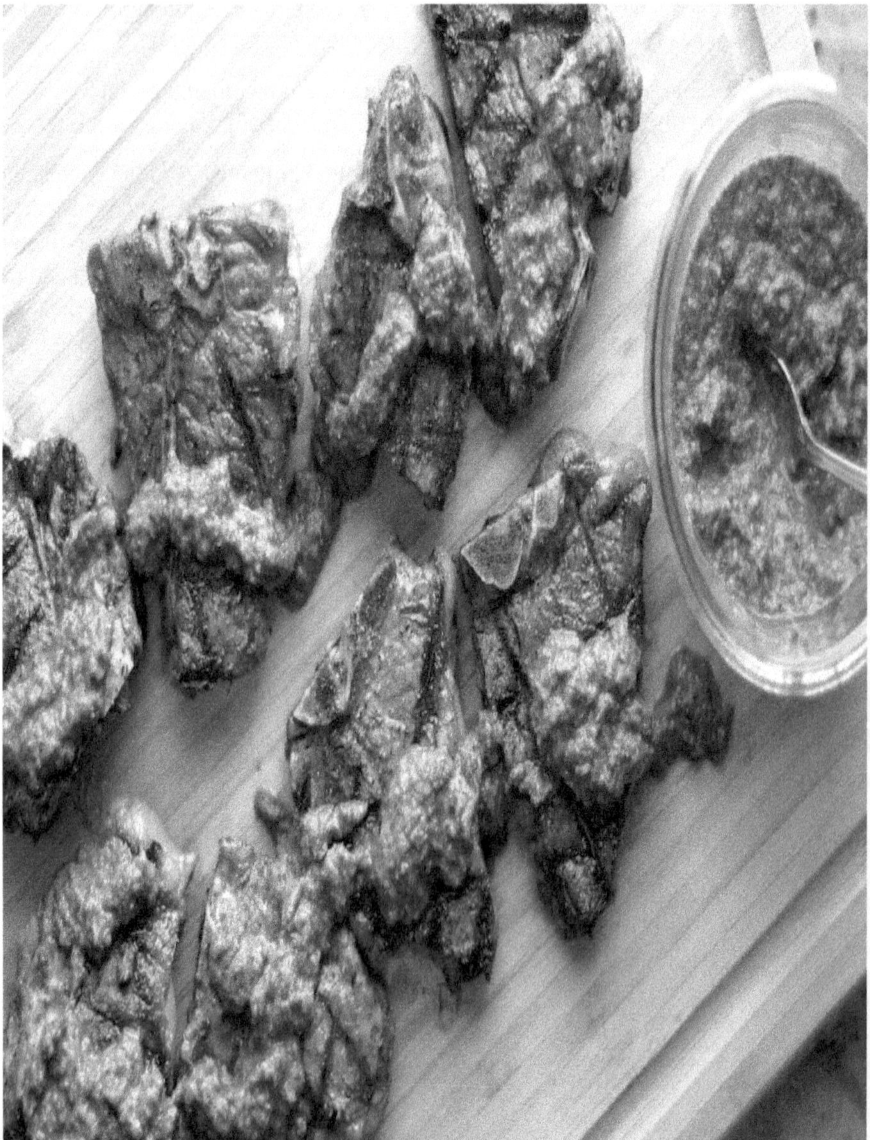

Servings: 4

Ingredients:

8 (4-ounce) lamb rib chops, trimmed of all visible fat

1⁄2 cup orange juice

1 garlic clove, crushed through a press

2 tablespoons chopped fresh mint, divided

2 large navel oranges

1 jalapeño, seeded and minced

1 tablespoon minced red onion

1 teaspoon extra virgin olive oil

1⁄4 teaspoon kosher salt

1⁄4 teaspoon freshly ground pepper

1⁄2 teaspoon canola oil

Directions:

1. Combine the lamb, orange juice, garlic, and 1 tablespoon of the mint in a large resealable plastic bag. Seal the bag and refrigerate 4 hours and up to 8 hours, turning the bag occasionally.
2. Cut a thin slice from the top and bottom of the oranges, exposing the flesh. Stand each orange upright, and using a sharp knife, thickly cut off the peel, following the contour of the fruit and removing all the white pith and membrane. Holding the oranges over a bowl, carefully cut along both sides of each section to free it from the membrane. Discard any seeds and let the sections fall into the bowl. Break the sections into small bits using two forks. Stir in the jalapeño, onion, remaining 1 tablespoon mint, and the olive oil.
3. Remove the lamb from the marinade and discard the marinade. Pat the lamb dry with paper towels and sprinkle with the salt and pepper.
4. Prepare the grill or heat a large grill pan over medium-high heat. Brush the grill rack or grill pan with the canola oil. Place the chops on the grill rack or in the grill pan and grill, turning once, 2 minutes on each side for medium- rare, or to the desired degree of doneness. Divide the chops and relish evenly among 4 plates and serve at once.

Nutrition Info:

15 g carb, 239 cal, 9 g fat, 3 g sat fat, 93 mg chol, 3 g fib, 25 g pro, 116 mg sod • Carb Choices: 1; Exchanges: 1 fruit, 3 lean protein

Yeast-risen Cornmeal Loaf

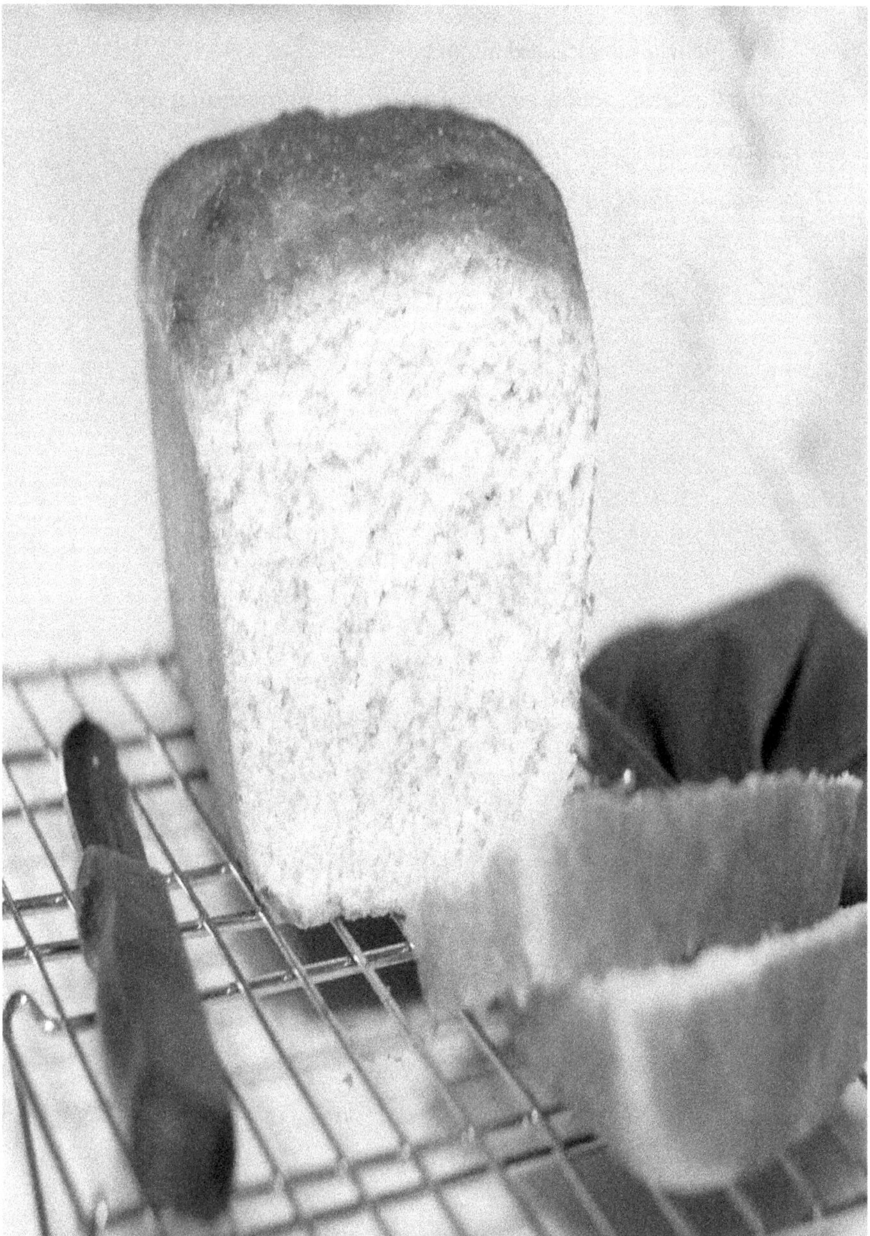

Servings: 12

Ingredients:

3⁄4 cup lukewarm water

1 package active dry yeast

1 1⁄4 to 1 1⁄2 cups unbleached all-purpose flour

1⁄2 cup fine-grind yellow cornmeal plus cornmeal for dusting pan

1 teaspoon salt

1 teaspoon canola oil

Directions:

1. Combine the water and yeast in a large bowl and stir until the yeast dissolves. Let stand 5 minutes. Add 1 1⁄4 cups of the flour, the cornmeal, and salt and stir until a soft dough forms.
2. Turn the dough out onto a lightly floured surface. Knead until smooth and elastic, about 8 minutes. Add enough of the remaining 1⁄4 cup flour, 1 tablespoon at a time, to prevent the dough from sticking to your hands. (Alternatively, knead the dough for 5 minutes at low speed with an electric mixer using a dough hook, adding enough of the remaining 1⁄4 cup flour, 1 tablespoon at a time, to make a smooth dough.)
3. Brush a large bowl with the oil. Place the dough in the bowl and turn to coat the top. Cover and let rise in a warm place (85°F), free from drafts, until doubled in size, about 1 hour.
4. Line a large baking sheet with parchment paper and dust the parchment lightly with cornmeal. Shape the dough into a 12 x 4-inch rectangle and place on the prepared baking sheet. Cover loosely with lightly oiled plastic wrap and let rise in a warm place (85°F), free from drafts, until doubled in size, about 45 minutes.
5. Preheat the oven to 400°F. Remove the plastic wrap and bake until the loaf is golden brown and sounds hollow when tapped, 20 to 25 minutes.
6. Remove the loaf from the pan and cool completely on a wire rack. Slice using a serrated knife. The bread can be stored inside a paper bag at room temperature for up to 2 days or frozen for up to 3 months.

Nutrition Info:

16 g carb, 80 cal, 1 g fat, 0 g sat fat, 0 mg chol, 1 g fib, 2 g pro, 197 mg sod • Carb Choices: 1; Exchanges: 1 starch

Muffuletta-style Roast Beef Sandwiches

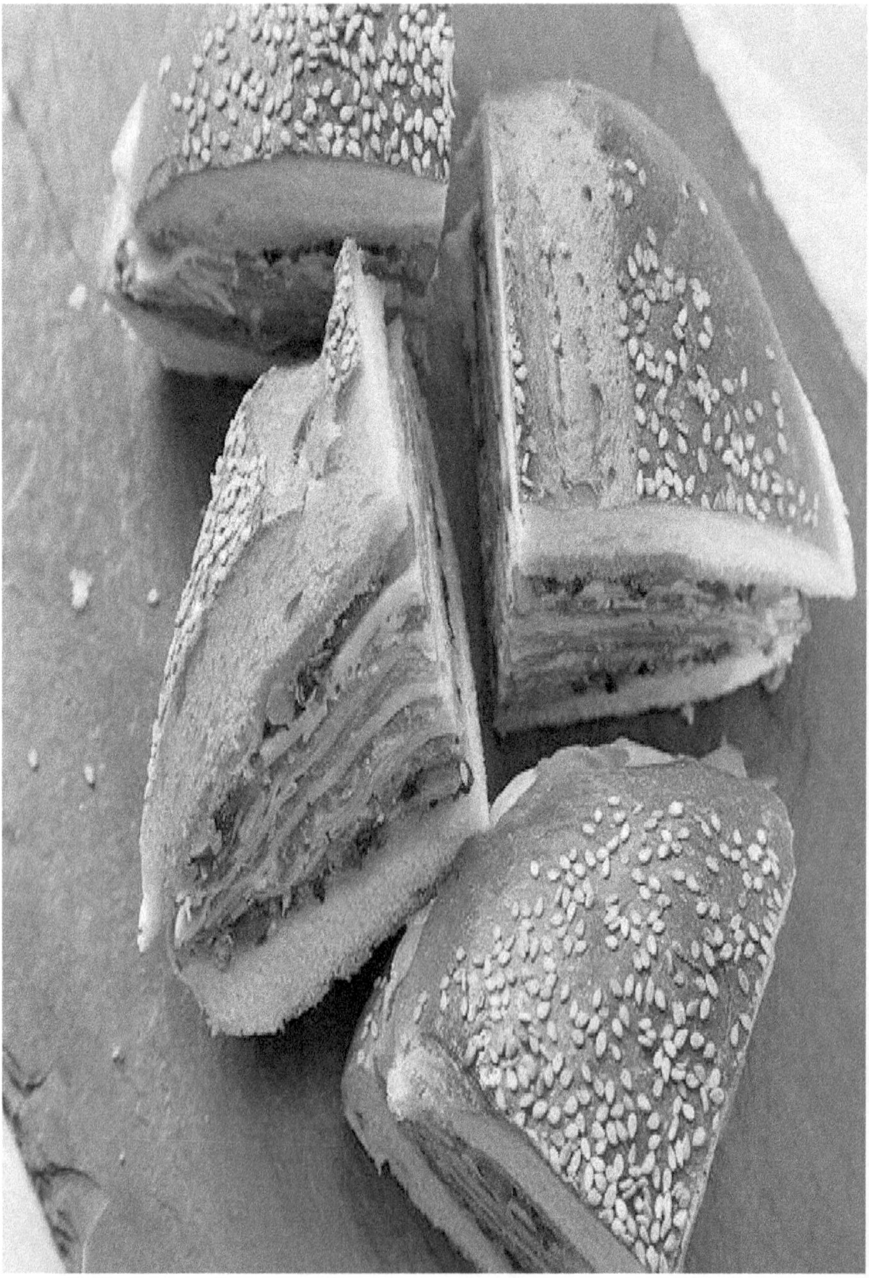

Servings: 4

Ingredients:

1⁄4 cup pimento-stuffed green olives, finely chopped

1⁄4 cup red Roasted Bell Peppers or roasted red peppers from a jar, finely chopped

1⁄4 cup diced celery

1 tablespoon chopped fresh Italian parsley

1 teaspoon red wine vinegar

1 teaspoon extra virgin olive oil

1 small garlic clove, minced

1⁄4 teaspoon dried oregano

1 (8-ounce) loaf whole wheat ciabatta

8 ounces thinly sliced rare roast beef

4 (1⁄2-ounce) slices Swiss cheese

2 plum tomatoes, thinly sliced

11⁄2 cups thinly sliced romaine lettuce or fresh spinach

Directions:

1. Stir together the olives, roasted peppers, celery, parsley, vinegar, oil, garlic, and oregano in a small bowl.
2. Cut the ciabatta in half crosswise, then cut each piece in half lengthwise. Remove and discard the soft inner crumbs from each piece of bread. Spread half of the olive mixture on the bottom halves of the bread. Top evenly with the beef and Swiss cheese, then with the remaining half of the olive mixture. Top with the tomatoes and lettuce. Cover with the top half of each piece of bread. Cut each sandwich in half and serve at once.

Nutrition Info:

28 g carb, 314 cal, 11 g fat, 4 g sat fat, 44 mg chol, 2 g fib, 25 g pro, 452 mg sod • Carb Choices: 2; Exchanges: 2 starch, 1 veg, 2 lean protein, 1 fat

Chocolate Souffle

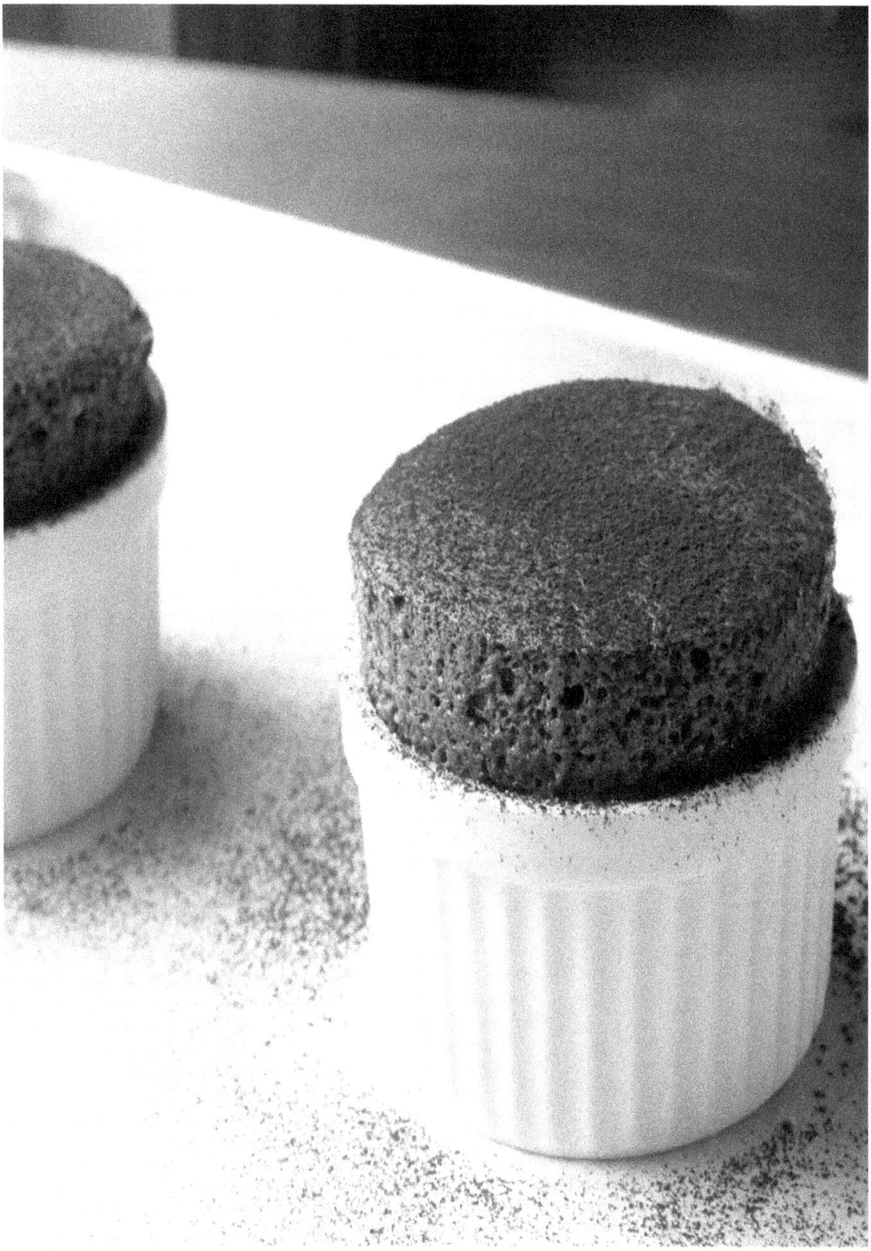

Servings: 10

Ingredients:

3⁄4 cup 1% low-fat milk

3⁄4 cup granulated sugar

1⁄2 cup unsweetened cocoa

3 tablespoons unbleached all-purpose flour

1⁄4 teaspoon salt

3 large eggs, separated

2 teaspoons vanilla extract

1 teaspoon unsalted butter, softened

1 large egg white

1⁄8 teaspoon cream of tartar

1 teaspoon confectioners' sugar

Directions:

1. Combine the milk, granulated sugar, cocoa, flour, and salt in a medium saucepan and whisk until smooth. Cook over medium heat, whisking constantly, until the mixture comes to a boil and thickens, about 5 minutes. Transfer the mixture to a large bowl and let stand 15 minutes to cool slightly. Whisk in the egg yolks and vanilla.
2. Preheat the oven to 350°F. Brush a 11⁄2-quart round baking dish with the butter.
3. Place the egg whites and cream of tartar in a large bowl and beat at high speed with an electric mixer until stiff peaks form. Fold the egg white mixture into the chocolate mixture in three additions, mixing until no white streaks remain.
4. Spoon the batter into the prepared baking dish. Bake until the soufflé is puffed and set, 35 to 40 minutes. Sprinkle the soufflé with the confectioners' sugar and serve at once.

Nutrition Info:

20 g carb, 113 cal, 3 g fat, 1 g sat fat, 65 mg chol, 1 g fib, 4 g pro, 94 mg sod • Carb Choices: 1; Exchanges: 1 carb, 1⁄2 fat

Swedish Meatballs

Servings: 4

Ingredients:

2 slices rye sandwich bread, each cut into 4 pieces

1 pound 95% lean ground beef

2 tablespoons minced onion

2 garlic cloves, minced

1 large egg white

3⁄4 teaspoon kosher salt, divided

1⁄4 teaspoon freshly ground pepper, divided

1⁄4 teaspoon ground nutmeg, divided

2 teaspoons extra virgin olive oil

1 1⁄2 cups Chicken Stock or low-sodium chicken broth

1 1⁄2 tablespoons unbleached all-purpose flour

1⁄2 cup plain low-fat Greek yogurt or strained yogurt

2 tablespoons chopped fresh Italian parsley

Directions:

1. Place the bread in a food processor and process until fine crumbs form (you should have about 1 cup).
2. Combine the breadcrumbs, beef, onion, garlic, egg white, 1⁄4 teaspoon of the salt, 1⁄8 teaspoon of the pepper, and 1⁄8 teaspoon of the nutmeg in a large bowl and mix thoroughly with your hands. Shape the mixture into about 32 (1-inch) meatballs.
3. Heat a large nonstick skillet over medium-high heat. Add the oil and tilt the pan to coat the bottom evenly. Add the meatballs in batches and cook, turning often, until no longer pink in the centers, 6 to 8 minutes. Transfer to a plate.
4. Whisk together the broth and flour in a medium bowl until smooth. Add the broth mixture to the pan and cook, whisking often, until the mixture comes to a boil and thickens, about 3 minutes. Stir in the remaining 1⁄2 teaspoon salt, 1⁄8 teaspoon pepper, and 1⁄8 teaspoon nutmeg.
5. Return the meatballs to the skillet and cook until heated through, about 2 minutes. Reduce the heat to low. Stir in the yogurt and cook, stirring constantly, just until heated through (do not boil). Remove from the heat and stir in the parsley. Divide the meatballs and sauce evenly among 4 shallow bowls and serve at once.

Nutrition Info:

10 g carb, 253 cal, 9 g fat, 4g sat fat, 74 mg chol, 1 g fib, 31 g pro, 455 mg sod • Carb Choices: 1; Exchanges: 1 starch, 3 lean protein, 1⁄2 fat

Tuna Tartines

Servings: 4

Ingredients:

2 (5-ounce) cans low-sodium chunk white albacore tuna in water, drained and flaked

6 Kalamata or niçoise olives, pitted and chopped

2 tablespoons chopped fresh Italian parsley

1 thin scallion, thinly sliced

2 teaspoons grated lemon zest

2 tablespoons lemon juice

1⁄4 teaspoon freshly ground pepper

1 tablespoon mayonnaise

1 tablespoon plain low-fat yogurt

2 (6-inch) whole wheat French rolls, cut in half lengthwise and toasted

1 1⁄2 cups loosely packed baby arugula

2 plum tomatoes, thinly sliced

Directions:

1. Combine the tuna, olives, parsley, scallion, lemon zest, lemon juice, and pepper in a medium bowl and toss gently to coat.
2. Stir together the mayonnaise and yogurt in a small bowl. Spread the mixture evenly on the cut sides of the rolls. Top evenly with the arugula, the tomatoes, and the tuna mixture. Serve at once.

Nutrition Info:

15 g carb, 200 cal, 7 g fat, 1 g sat fat, 23 mg chol, 2 g fib, 21 g pro, 280 mg sod • Carb Choices: 1; Exchanges: 1 starch, 3 lean protein, 1 fat

Citrus Spice Rub

Servings: About 2 Teaspoons

Ingredients:

2 teaspoons extra virgin olive oil

2 teaspoons grated lemon zest

1 teaspoon grated lime zest

1 garlic clove, crushed through a press

1 teaspoon ground cumin

1 teaspoon ground coriander

1 teaspoon paprika

1/2 teaspoon kosher salt

1/8 teaspoon freshly ground pepper

Directions:

1. Stir together all the ingredients in a small bowl.

Nutrition Info:

1 g carb, 27 cal, 3 g fat, 0 g sat fat, 0 mg chol, 1 g fib, 0 g pro, 142 mg sod • Carb Choices: 0; Exchanges: 1⁄2 fat

Cilantro Chicken Salad Wraps

Servings: 4

Ingredients:

2 tablespoons mayonnaise

2 tablespoons plain low-fat yogurt

1/2 teaspoon grated lime zest

1tablespoon lime juice

1 jalapeño, seeded and minced

1 small garlic clove, minced

1/8 teaspoon ground cumin

1/2 teaspoon kosher salt

12 ounces chopped cooked chicken breast (about 2 cups)

2 tablespoons minced red onion

2 tablespoons chopped fresh cilantro

4 (8-inch) whole wheat flour tortillas

4 large leaves leaf lettuce

2 plum tomatoes, thinly sliced

Directions:

1. Stir together the mayonnaise, yogurt, lime zest, lime juice, jalapeño, garlic, cumin, and salt in a medium bowl. Add the chicken, onion, and cilantro and stir to mix well.
2. Top each of the tortillas with a lettuce leaf, then top the lettuce evenly with the tomato slices. Top evenly with the chicken mixture and roll up. Cut each roll in half.

Nutrition Info:

26 g carb, 359 cal, 13 g fat, 3 g sat fat, 75 mg chol, 6 g fib, 32 g pro, 607 mg sod • Carb Choices: 2; Exchanges: 1 1/2 starch, 1 veg, 2 fat

Basil-crusted Fish Fillets with Roasted Cherry Tomatoes

Servings: 4

Ingredients:

TOMATOES

2 cups grape tomatoes

2 teaspoons extra virgin olive oil

1 tablespoon sherry vinegar or white wine vinegar

1 tablespoon capers, rinsed and drained

1⁄8 teaspoon kosher salt

1⁄8 teaspoon freshly ground pepper

2 tablespoons chopped fresh basil

FISH

4 (5-ounce) thick white-fleshed fish fillets

1⁄4 teaspoon kosher salt

1⁄8 teaspoon freshly ground pepper

2 tablespoons chopped fresh basil

2 teaspoons extra virgin olive oil

Directions:

1. To make the tomatoes, preheat the oven to 400°F.
2. Combine the tomatoes and oil in a medium baking dish and stir to coat. Bake until some of the tomatoes begin to burst, 18 to 20 minutes.
3. Transfer the tomatoes and any pan juices to a medium bowl. Stir in the vinegar, capers, salt, and pepper. Stir in the basil just before serving. Serve warm or at room temperature.
4. Meanwhile, to make the fish, sprinkle the fillets with the salt and pepper, then with the basil, pressing to adhere.
5. Heat a large nonstick skillet over medium heat. Add the oil and tilt the pan to coat the bottom evenly. Add the fillets and cook, turning once, until the fish flakes easily with a fork, about 4 minutes on each side. Divide the fish and tomatoes among 4 plates and serve at once.

Nutrition Info:

3 g carb, 160 cal, 6 g fat, 1 g sat fat, 54 mg chol, 1 g fib, 23 g pro, 249 mg sod • Carb Choices: 0; Exchanges: 1 veg, 3 lean protein, 1 fat

Asian Edamame And Radish Salad

Servings: 4

Ingredients:

2 cups frozen shelled edamame

1 1⁄2 tablespoons canola oil

1 tablespoon rice vinegar

1 tablespoon lime juice

1 tablespoon reduced-sodium soy sauce

1⁄2 teaspoon kosher salt

1⁄4 teaspoon Asian sesame oil

2 teaspoons minced fresh ginger

6 radishes, thinly sliced

1⁄2 cup diced yellow or green bell pepper

1⁄2 cup diced hothouse (English) cucumber

1⁄4 cup chopped fresh cilantro or 2 tablespoons chopped fresh mint

Directions:

1. Bring a medium saucepan of water to a boil over high heat. Add the edamame and cook until tender, about 5 minutes. Drain in a colander and rinse with cold running water until cool.
2. Meanwhile, whisk together the canola oil, vinegar, lime juice, soy sauce, salt, sesame oil, and ginger in a large bowl. Add the edamame, radishes, bell pepper, cucumber, and cilantro and stir to combine. Serve the salad at room temperature or chilled. The salad tastes best on the day it is made, but it can be refrigerated, covered, for up to 2 days.

Nutrition Info:

7 g carb, 125 cal, 8 g fat, 0 g sat fat, 0 mg chol, 3 g fib, 7 g pro, 299 mg sod • Carb Choices: 1⁄2; Exchanges: 1⁄2 carb, 1 plant-based protein, 1 fat

Ropa Vieja Tacos

Servings: 8

Ingredients:

2 pounds flank steak, trimmed of all visible fat

1⁄2 teaspoon kosher salt

1⁄4 teaspoon freshly ground pepper

4 teaspoons extra virgin olive oil, divided

1 large onion, thinly sliced

1 large green bell pepper, thinly sliced

1 large red bell pepper, thinly sliced

2 garlic cloves, minced

2 teaspoons chili powder

1 teaspoon ground cumin

1 teaspoon dried oregano

1⁄4 teaspoon ground cayenne

1 (141⁄2-ounce) can no-salt-added diced tomatoes

1⁄4 cup pimento-stuffed green olives, sliced

2 tablespoons no-salt-added tomato paste

16 (6-inch) whole wheat flour tortillas, warmed

1 cup Winter Tomato Salsa or purchased salsa

Chopped fresh cilantro

Lime wedges

Directions:

1. Cut the steak crosswise into 3-inch pieces. Sprinkle the steak with the salt and pepper. Heat a Dutch oven over medium-high heat. Add 2 teaspoons of the oil and tilt the pan to coat the bottom evenly. Add half of the steak and cook, turning to brown on both sides, 6 to 8 minutes. Transfer to a plate. Repeat with the remaining steak (additional oil should not be necessary). Return the steak to the pot and add water to cover. Bring to a boil. Reduce the heat to low, cover, and simmer until the steak is very tender, adding additional water, if necessary, to keep the steak almost covered, about 1 1⁄2 hours.
2. Transfer the steak to a plate. Increase the heat to high and cook the liquid, uncovered, until reduced to 2 cups. Shred the beef using 2 forks and set aside.
3. Meanwhile, heat a large nonstick skillet over medium-high heat. Add the remaining 2 teaspoons oil and tilt the pan to coat the bottom evenly. Add the onion and bell peppers and cook, stirring often, until the vegetables are softened, 8 minutes. Add the garlic, chili powder, cumin, oregano, and cayenne and cook, stirring constantly, until fragrant, 30 seconds. Add the 2 cups of cooking liquid, the shredded beef, tomatoes, olives, and tomato paste and bring to a boil. Reduce the heat to low, cover, and simmer until the peppers are tender, 10 minutes. Uncover and simmer until the stew is thickened, 5 to 10 minutes longer.
4. Serve the stew in the tortillas, topped with the salsa and cilantro with the lime wedges alongside. The stew can be frozen for up to 3 months.

Nutrition Info:

33 g carb, 392 cal, 16 g fat, 4 g sat fat, 48 mg chol, 18 g fib, 27 g pro, 730 mg sod • Carb Choices: 1 1⁄2; Exchanges: 1 starch, 1 veg, 3 lean protein, 1 1⁄2 fat

Roasted Beets with Apple-walnut Dressing

Servings: 4

Ingredients:

1⁄2 cup apple cider

1 teaspoon apple cider vinegar

1⁄2 teaspoon kosher salt, divided

Pinch of freshly ground pepper

1 tablespoon walnut oil or extra virgin olive oil

1 recipe Foil-Roasted Beets or Basic Boiled Beets

2 teaspoons extra virgin olive oil

2 tablespoons walnuts, toasted and chopped

Directions:

1. To make the dressing, place the cider in a small skillet and bring to a boil over high heat. Reduce the heat to low and simmer, uncovered, until the cider is thickened and reduced to about 2 tablespoons, 6 minutes. Transfer to a medium bowl and allow to cool.
2. Whisk in the vinegar, 1⁄4 teaspoon of the salt, and the pepper. Slowly whisk in the walnut oil.
3. Cut the beets into bite-size pieces.
4. Heat a large nonstick skillet over medium-high heat. Add the olive oil and tilt the pan to coat the bottom evenly. Add the beets and remaining 1⁄4 teaspoon salt and cook, stirring occasionally, until the beets are lightly browned, 6 minutes. Add the beets to the dressing and toss gently to coat.
5. To serve, spoon the beets onto a serving platter and sprinkle with the walnuts. Serve hot or warm.

Nutrition Info:

11 g carb, 119 cal, 8 g fat, 1 g sat fat, 0 mg chol, 2 g fib, 2 g pro, 133 mg sod • Carb Choices: 1; Exchanges: 1⁄2 carb, 1 veg, 1 1⁄2 fat

Fennel Gratin

Servings: 4

Ingredients:

2 large bulbs fennel

1 teaspoon extra virgin olive oil

1⁄2 teaspoon kosher salt

Pinch of freshly ground pepper

1 ounce freshly grated Parmesan (about 1⁄4 cup)

Directions:

1. Preheat the oven to 400°F.
2. Trim the tough outer stalks from the fennel bulbs. Cut each one in half vertically and discard the cores. Cut each half lengthwise into 1⁄2-inch slices.
3. In a saucepan fitted with a steamer basket, bring 1 inch of water to a boil over high heat. Add the fennel, reduce the heat to low, cover, and steam until tender, about 5 minutes.
4. Place the fennel in a shallow 2-quart baking dish. Drizzle with the oil, sprinkle with the salt and pepper, and toss to coat. Arrange the fennel evenly in the dish and sprinkle with the Parmesan.
5. Bake, uncovered, until the cheese is melted, 15 to 20 minutes. Serve hot or warm.

Nutrition Info:

9 g carb, 68 cal, 3 g fat, 1 g sat fat, 4 mg chol, 4 g fib, 3 g pro, 277 mg sod • Carb Choices: 1⁄2; Exchanges: 2 veg, 1⁄2 fat

Wheat Berry–mango Salad

Servings: 6

Ingredients:

1 cup wheat berries, farro, kamut, or spelt

4 cups water

3⁄4 teaspoon kosher salt, divided

1 teaspoon grated lemon zest

1⁄4 cup lemon juice

1 tablespoon extra virgin olive oil

1 tablespoon honey

1⁄2 teaspoon ground cumin

1⁄2 teaspoon ground coriander

1⁄8 teaspoon freshly ground pepper

1 mango, peeled, pitted, and chopped

1⁄4 cup diced carrot

2 tablespoons minced red onion

2 tablespoons chopped fresh Italian parsley

3 tablespoons slivered almonds, toasted

Directions:

1. Combine the wheat berries, water, and 1⁄2 teaspoon of the salt in a medium saucepan and bring to a boil over high heat. Reduce the heat to low, cover, and simmer until tender yet firm to the bite, 45 minutes to 1 hour. Drain.
2. Meanwhile, whisk together the lemon zest, lemon juice, oil, honey, cumin, coriander, remaining 1⁄4 teaspoon salt, and the pepper in a large bowl. Stir in the hot cooked wheat berries and let stand to cool to room temperature, stirring occasionally. Stir in the mango, carrot, onion, and parsley. Stir in the almonds just before serving. Serve the salad at room temperature or chilled. The salad tastes best on the day it is made, but it can be refrigerated for up to 2 days.

Nutrition Info:

32 g carb, 188 cal, 5 g fat, 0 g sat fat, 0 mg chol, 4 g fib, 6 g pro, 146 mg sod • Carb Choices: 2; Exchanges: 11⁄2 starch, 1⁄2 carb, 1 fat

Roasted Broccoli with Balsamic-dijon Vinaigrette

Servings: 4

Ingredients:

5 cups broccoli florets, cut into bite-size pieces

1 teaspoon plus 1 tablespoon extra virgin olive oil, divided

2 teaspoons balsamic vinegar

1⁄2 teaspoon Dijon mustard

1⁄4 teaspoon kosher salt

Pinch of freshly ground pepper

Directions:

1. Preheat the oven to 425°F.
2. Place the broccoli in a medium roasting pan. Drizzle with 1 teaspoon of the oil and toss to coat. Bake, stirring once, until the broccoli is lightly browned and tender, about 15 minutes.
3. Meanwhile, whisk together the vinegar, mustard, salt, and pepper in a medium bowl. Slowly whisk in the remaining 1 tablespoon oil. Add the broccoli to the bowl and toss to coat. Serve at once.

Nutrition Info:

5 g carb, 66 cal, 5 g fat, 1 g sat fat, 0 mg chol, 3 g fib, 3 g pro, 110 mg sod • Carb Choices: 0; Exchanges: 1 veg, 1 fat

Coconut Shrimp Soup with Basmati Rice

Servings: 4

Ingredients:

2 teaspoons canola oil

1 small red bell pepper, cut into short, thin strips

1 small onion, halved and sliced

2 tablespoons minced fresh ginger

2 garlic cloves, minced

21⁄2 cups Chicken Stock or low-sodium chicken broth

1 (131⁄2-ounce) can reduced-fat coconut milk

1 tablespoon green curry paste

1-pound medium peeled deveined shrimp

2 tablespoons lime juice

2 cups hot cooked brown basmati rice

Thinly sliced scallions

Thinly sliced fresh basil leaves

Directions:

1. Heat a large pot over medium heat. Add the oil and tilt the pot to evenly coat the bottom. Add the bell pepper and onion and cook, stirring often, until the vegetables are softened, 5 minutes. Add the ginger and garlic and cook, stirring constantly, until fragrant, 30 seconds.
2. Add the stock, coconut milk, and curry paste and bring to a boil. Add the shrimp and cook until the shrimp turn pink, 2 minutes. Remove from the heat and stir in the lime juice. Spoon 1⁄2 cup of the rice into each of 4 bowls and ladle the soup evenly over the rice. Sprinkle each serving with scallions and basil and serve at once. The soup is best when eaten immediately.

Nutrition Info:

23 g carb, 264 cal, 10 g fat, 6 g sat fat, 171 mg chol, 2 g fib, 24 g pro, 375 mg sod • Carb Choices: 11⁄2; Exchanges: 1 starch, 1 veg, 3 lean protein, 1 fat

Rosemary-olive Focaccia

Servings: 15

Ingredients:

1 cup lukewarm water

1 package active dry yeast

1 1⁄4 cups unbleached all-purpose flour, divided

1 cup whole wheat flour

3⁄4 teaspoon salt

2 teaspoons extra virgin olive oil, divided

1⁄3 cup Kalamata olives, pitted and sliced

2 teaspoons chopped fresh rosemary or 1⁄2 teaspoon crumbled dried rosemary

Directions:

1. Combine the water and yeast in a large bowl and stir until the yeast dissolves. Let stand 5 minutes. Add 1 cup of the all-purpose flour, the whole wheat flour, and salt and stir until a soft dough forms.
2. Turn the dough out onto a lightly floured surface. Knead until smooth and elastic, about 8 minutes. Add enough of the remaining 1⁄4 cup all-purpose flour, 1 tablespoon at a time, to prevent the dough from sticking to your hands. (Alternatively, knead the dough for 5 minutes at low speed with an electric mixer using a dough hook, adding enough of the remaining 1⁄4 cup all-purpose flour, 1 tablespoon at a time, to make a smooth dough.)
3. Brush a large bowl with 1 teaspoon of the oil. Place the dough in the bowl and turn to coat the top. Cover and let rise in a warm place (85°F), free from drafts, until doubled in size, about 1 hour.
4. Brush a 15 x 10-inch jellyroll pan or large rimmed baking sheet with the remaining 1 teaspoon oil. Place the dough into the pan and pat to evenly cover the pan. If you have trouble stretching the dough, let it rest 5 minutes, then try again.
5. Sprinkle the dough evenly with the olives and rosemary. Cover loosely with lightly oiled plastic wrap and let rise in a warm place (85°F), free from drafts, until doubled in size, about 45 minutes.
6. Preheat the oven to 400°F. Remove the plastic wrap and bake until the focaccia is lightly browned, 25 to 30 minutes. Transfer the focaccia to a cutting board and cut into 15 pieces. Serve warm or at room temperature. The bread is best the day it is made.

Nutrition Info:

14 g carb, 78 cal, 1 g fat, 0 g sat fat, 0 mg chol, 1 g fib, 3 g pro, 149 mg sod • Carb Choices: 1; Exchanges: 1 starch

Italian Tofu

Servings: 4

Ingredients:

2 cups Marinara Sauce

1 large egg white

2 tablespoons water

2⁄3 cup panko crumbs

1⁄4 cup plus 2 tablespoons freshly grated Parmesan, divided

1⁄4 teaspoon dried oregano

1⁄4 teaspoon dried basil

1⁄8 teaspoon freshly ground pepper

1 (1-pound) package firm reduced-fat tofu, cut crosswise into 8 slices

4 teaspoons extra virgin olive oil, divided

Directions:

1. Heat the sauce in a saucepan over medium heat until hot, if necessary.
2. Place the egg white and water in a shallow dish and beat lightly with a fork. Stir together the panko crumbs, 1⁄4 cup of the Parmesan, the oregano, basil, and pepper in another shallow dish. Dip the tofu, 1 slice at a time, into the egg white mixture, then into the crumb mixture, pressing to adhere the crumbs.
3. Heat a large nonstick skillet over medium heat. Add 2 teaspoons of the oil and tilt the pan to coat the bottom evenly. Add 4 slices of the tofu and cook, turning once, until the crumbs are lightly browned, 6 to 8 minutes. Transfer to a plate keep warm. Repeat with the remaining oil and tofu.
4. Divide the tofu among 4 plates, top with the sauce and the remaining 2 tablespoons Parmesan. Serve at once.

Nutrition Info:

20 g carb, 269 cal, 14 g fat, 2 g sat fat, 7 mg chol, 4 g fib, 19 g pro, 222 mg sod • Carb Choices: 1; Exchanges: 1⁄2 starch, 1 veg, 2 plant- based protein, 1 fat

Balsamic Vinaigrette

Servings: 1⁄3 Cup

Ingredients:

3 tablespoons extra virgin olive oil

2 tablespoons balsamic vinegar

1 tablespoon minced shallots

1 teaspoon honey

1⁄2 teaspoon Dijon mustard

1⁄4 teaspoon kosher salt

1⁄8 teaspoon freshly ground pepper

Directions:

1. Whisk together all the ingredients in a small bowl. The dressing can be refrigerated, covered, for up to 3 days.

Nutrition Info:

2 g carb, 54 cal, 5 g fat, 1 g sat fat, 0 mg chol, 0 g fib, 0 g pro, 39 mg sod • Carb Choices: 0; Exchanges: 1 fat

Rosemary Roasted Pork Tenderloin

Servings: 4

Ingredients:

1⁄2 teaspoon canola oil

1 (1-pound) pork tenderloin, trimmed of all visible fat

1⁄2 teaspoon kosher salt

1⁄4 teaspoon freshly ground pepper

1 tablespoon real maple syrup

1 1⁄2 tablespoons chopped fresh rosemary or 1 teaspoon crumbled dried rosemary

Directions:

1. Preheat the oven to 400°F. Line a rimmed baking sheet with foil and brush the foil with the oil.
2. Sprinkle the tenderloin with the salt and pepper. Brush the maple syrup over the tenderloin. Sprinkle with the rosemary, pressing to adhere to the pork.
3. Place on the prepared baking sheet and bake, turning once, until an instant-read thermometer inserted into the center of the tenderloin reads 145°F, 15 to 20 minutes. Cover loosely with foil and let stand about 10 minutes. Cut the tenderloin into thin slices, divide evenly among 4 plates, and serve at once.

Nutrition Info:

4 g carb, 151 cal, 4 g fat, 1 g sat fat, 63 mg chol, 0 g fib, 23 g pro, 185 mg sod • Carb Choices: 0; Exchanges: 3 lean protein

Brussels Sprouts with Caraway

Servings: 6

Ingredients:

1 tablespoon extra virgin olive oil

1 small onion, halved and thinly sliced

1⁄2 teaspoon caraway seeds

1 pound Brussels sprouts, trimmed and quartered

1⁄2 cup Chicken Stock or low-sodium chicken broth

1⁄2 teaspoon kosher salt

1⁄8 teaspoon freshly ground pepper

Directions:

1. Heat a large nonstick skillet over medium heat. Add the oil and tilt the pan to coat the bottom evenly. Add the onion and caraway seeds and cook, stirring occasionally, until the onion is tender, 5 minutes.
2. Add the Brussels sprouts, stock, salt, and pepper. Cover and cook, stirring often, until the Brussels sprouts are crisp-tender, about 5 minutes. If excess liquid remains in the pan, uncover and cook until most of the liquid evaporates. Spoon the Brussels sprouts into a serving bowl and serve at once.

Nutrition Info:

7 g carb, 50 cal, 2 g fat, 0 g sat fat, 0 mg chol, 3 g fib, 3 g pro, 122 mg sod • Carb Choices: 1; Exchanges: 1 vegetable

Alphabetical Index

CPSIA information can be obtained
at www.ICGtesting.com
Printed in the USA
LVHW050250090621
689715LV00011B/675

9 781803 100319